T0348620

Gastroparesis: Current Opinions and New Endoscopic Therapies

Editors

HUIMIN CHEN
QIANG CAI

GASTROINTESTINAL ENDOSCOPY CLINICS OF NORTH AMERICA

www.giendo.theclinics.com

Consulting Editor
CHARLES J. LIGHTDALE

January 2019 • Volume 29 • Number 1

ELSEVIER

1600 John F. Kennedy Boulevard • Suite 1800 • Philadelphia, Pennsylvania, 19103-2899

http://www.theclinics.com

GASTROINTESTINAL ENDOSCOPY CLINICS OF NORTH AMERICA Volume 29, Number 1
January 2019 ISSN 1052-5157, ISBN-13: 978-0-323-65465-4

Editor: Kerry Holland
Developmental Editor: Donald Mumford

Gastrointestinal Endoscopy Clinics of North America (ISSN 1052-5157) is published quarterly by Elsevier Inc., 360 Park Avenue South, New York, NY 10010-1710. Months of issue are January, April, July, and October. Business and Editorial Offices: 1600 John F. Kennedy Blvd., Suite 1800, Philadelphia, PA, 19103-2899. Periodicals postage paid at New York, NY and additional mailing offices. Subscription prices are $359.00 per year for US individuals, $624.00 per year for US institutions, $100.00 per year for US students and residents, $399.00 per year for Canadian individuals, $737.00 per year for Canadian institutions, $476.00 per year for international individuals, $737.00 per year for international institutions, and $245.00 per year for Canadian and international students/residents. To receive student/resident rate, orders must be accompanied by name of affiliated institution, date of term, and the *signature* of program/residency coordinator on institution letterhead. Orders will be billed at individual rate until proof of status is received. Foreign air speed delivery is included in all *Clinics* subscription prices. All prices are subject to change without notice. **POSTMASTER:** Send address change to *Gastrointestinal Endoscopy Clinics of North America*, Elsevier Health Sciences Division, Subscription Customer Service, 3251 Riverport Lane, Maryland Heights, MO 63043. **Customer Service: 1-800-654-2452 (US). From outside the United States, call 1-314-447-8871. Fax: 1-314-447-8029. E-mail: JournalsCustomerService-usa@elsevier.com (for print support) or JournalsOnlineSupport-usa@elsevier.com (for online support).**

Reprints. For copies of 100 or more, of articles in this publication, please contact the Commercial Reprints Department, Elsevier Inc., 360 Park Avenue South, New York, NY 10010-1710. Tel. 212-633-3874; Fax: 212-633-3820; E-mail: reprints@elsevier.com.

Gastrointestinal Endoscopy Clinics of North America is covered in *Excerpta Medica, MEDLINE/PubMed (Index Medicus), and MEDLINE/MEDLARS.*

Contributors

CONSULTING EDITOR

CHARLES J. LIGHTDALE, MD
Professor of Medicine, Division of Digestive and Liver Diseases, Columbia University Medical Center, New York, New York, USA

EDITORS

HUIMIN CHEN, MD, PhD
Assistant Professor, Division of Digestive Diseases, Emory University School of Medicine, Atlanta, Georgia, USA; Attending Physician, Division of Gastroenterology and Hepatology, Renji Hospital, School of Medicine, Shanghai Jiaotong University, Shanghai, China

QIANG CAI, MD, PhD, FASGE, FACG
Professor of Medicine, Director, Advanced Endoscopy Fellowship, Division of Digestive Diseases, Emory University School of Medicine, Atlanta, Georgia, USA

AUTHORS

THOMAS L. ABELL, MD
The Arthur M. Schoen, MD, Chair in Gastroenterology, Department of Medicine, Division of Gastroenterology, Hepatology and Nutrition, University of Louisville, Louisville, Kentucky, USA

HADI ATASSI, DO
Department of Medicine, Division of Internal Medicine, University of Louisville, Louisville, Kentucky, USA

OLAYA I. BREWER GUTIERREZ, MD
Advanced Therapeutic Fellow, Division of Gastroenterology and Hepatology, The Johns Hopkins Hospital, Baltimore, Maryland, USA

QIANG CAI, MD, PhD, FASGE, FACG
Professor of Medicine, Director, Advanced Endoscopy Fellowship, Division of Digestive Diseases, Emory University School of Medicine, Atlanta, Georgia, USA

MICHAEL CAMILLERI, MD
Atherton and Winifred W. Bean Professor, Professor of Medicine, Pharmacology, and Physiology, Consultant, Division of Gastroenterology and Hepatology, Department of Medicine, Mayo Clinic College of Medicine and Science, Mayo Clinic, Rochester, Minnesota, USA

HUIMIN CHEN, MD, PhD
Assistant Professor, Division of Digestive Diseases, Emory University School of Medicine, Atlanta, Georgia, USA; Division of Gastroenterology and Hepatology, Renji Hospital, School of Medicine, Shanghai Jiaotong University, Shanghai, China

SUNIL DACHA, MD
Assistant Professor, Division of Digestive Diseases, Emory University School of Medicine, Atlanta, Georgia, USA

CHRISTY M. DUNST, MD, FACS
Division of GI/MIS, Esophageal Surgeon, Fellowship Program Director, The Oregon Clinic, Portland, Oregon, USA

MAHESH GAJENDRAN, MD, MPH, FACP
Department of Internal Medicine, Texas Tech University Health Sciences Center, Paul L. Foster School of Medicine, El Paso, Texas, USA

JAMES GALT, PhD
Department of Radiology and Imaging Sciences, Emory University School of Medicine, Atlanta, Georgia, USA

GUILLAUME GOURCEROL, MD, PhD
Professor of Medicine, Gastroenterology Department, Rouen University Hospital, Rouen, France

QUNYE GUAN, MD, PhD
Associate Professor, Division of Digestive Diseases, Emory University School of Medicine, Atlanta, Georgia, USA; Department of Gastroenterology, Weihai Municipal Hospital, Weihai, China

RAGHUVEER HALKAR, MD
Department of Radiology and Imaging Sciences, Emory University School of Medicine, Atlanta, Georgia, USA

JÉRÉMIE JACQUES, MD
Associate Professor, Gastroenterology Department, Limoges University Hospital, Rouen, France

MOUEN A. KHASHAB, MD
Associate Professor of Medicine, Director of Therapeutic Endoscopy, Division of Gastroenterology and Hepatology, The Johns Hopkins Hospital, Baltimore, Maryland, USA

BRIAN E. LACY, MD, PhD
Staff Physician, Division of Gastroenterology and Hepatology, Mayo Clinic, Jacksonville, Florida, USA

VLADIMIR LAMM, MD
Resident, Division of Digestive Diseases, Emory University, Atlanta, Georgia, USA

ROMAIN LEGROS, MD
Gastroenterology Department, Limoges University Hospital, Rouen, France

BAIWEN LI, MD, PhD
Associate Professor, Division of Digestive Diseases, Emory University School of Medicine, Atlanta, Georgia, USA; Department of Gastroenterology, Shanghai General Hospital, Shanghai Jiaotong University, Shanghai, China

PRIYADARSHINI LOGANATHAN, MD
Department of Internal Medicine, Texas Tech University Health Sciences Center, Paul L. Foster School of Medicine, El Paso, Texas, USA

HUI LUO, MD
Assistant Professor, Division of Digestive Diseases, Emory University School of Medicine, Atlanta, Georgia, USA; Department of Pancreatobiliary Disease, Xijing Hospital of Digestive Diseases, Fourth Military Medical University, Xi'an, China

RICHARD W. McCALLUM, FACP, FRACP (AUST), FACG, AGAF
Professor of Medicine and Founding Chair, Division of Gastroenterology, Texas Tech University Health Sciences Center, Paul L. Foster School of Medicine, El Paso, Texas, USA

PARIT MEKAROONKAMOL, MD
Assistant Professor, Division of Digestive Diseases, Emory University School of Medicine, Atlanta, Georgia, USA

JACQUES MONTEIL, MD, PhD
Professor of Medicine, Nuclear Medicine Department, Limoges University Hospital, Limoges, France

BAHA MOSHIREE, MD, MS-CI
Professor of Medicine, Division of Gastroenterology, University of North Carolina, Charlotte, North Carolina, USA

CHRISTOPHER M. NAVAS, MD
Resident Physician, Department of Internal Medicine, Dartmouth-Hitchcock Medical Center, Lebanon, New Hampshire, USA

PANKAJ J. PASRICHA, MD
Center for Neurogastroenterology, Vice-Chair of Medicine, Professor of Medicine and Neurosciences, Department of Medicine, Johns Hopkins School of Medicine, The Johns Hopkins Hospital, Baltimore, Maryland, USA

TRISHA S. PASRICHA, MD
Junior Assistant Resident, Osler Medical Training Program, Department of Medicine, The Johns Hopkins Hospital, Baltimore, Maryland, USA

NIHAL K. PATEL, MD
Fellow Physician, Section of Gastroenterology and Hepatology, Dartmouth-Hitchcock Medical Center, Lebanon, New Hampshire, USA

VAISHALI PATEL, MD, MHS
Assistant Professor, Division of Digestive Diseases, Emory University School of Medicine, Atlanta, Georgia, USA

MICHAEL POTTER, MD
Department of Gastroenterology, University of Newcastle, John Hunter Hospital, New Lambton Heights, New South Wales, Australia

DENIS SAUTEREAU, MD
Professor of Medicine, Gastroenterology Department, Limoges University Hospital, Rouen, France

SHANSHAN SHEN, MD, PhD
Assistant Professor, Division of Digestive Diseases, Emory University School of Medicine, Atlanta, Georgia, USA; Department of Gastroenterology, Nanjing Drum Tower Hospital, The Affiliated Hospital of Nanjing University Medical School, Nanjing, China

ROBERT M. SPANDORFER, MD
Department of Digestive Diseases, Emory University School of Medicine, Atlanta, Georgia, USA

LEE L. SWANSTRÖM, MD, FACS, FASGE, FRCSEng
Division of GI/MIS, Esophageal Surgeon, The Oregon Clinic, Clinical Professor of Surgery, Oregon Health & Science University, Portland, Oregon, USA; Scientific Director, IHU-Strasbourg, Strasbourg, France

LAWRENCE A. SZARKA, MD
Consultant, Division of Gastroenterology and Hepatology, Assistant Professor, Department of Medicine, Mayo Clinic College of Medicine and Science, Mayo Clinic, Rochester, Minnesota, USA

NICHOLAS J. TALLEY, MD, PhD
Pro-Vice Chancellor, Global Research, Digestive and Health Neurogastroenterology, New Lambton, Australia

JIE TAO, MD
Division of Digestive Diseases, Emory University School of Medicine, Atlanta, Georgia, USA; Department of Hepatobiliary Surgery, The First Affiliated Hospital of Xi'an Jiaotong University, Xi'an, China

CICILY T. VACHAPARAMBIL, MD
Resident, Division of Digestive Diseases, Emory University, Atlanta, Georgia, USA

JENNIFER XU, MD
Resident, Division of Digestive Diseases, Emory University, Atlanta, Georgia, USA

YIN ZHU, MD, PhD
Department of Gastroenterology, First Affiliated Hospital of Nanchang University, Nanchang City, Jiangxi, China

AHMED M. ZIHNI, MD, MPH
Division of GI/MIS, The Oregon Clinic, Portland Providence Cancer Center, Portland, Oregon, USA

Contents

Gastroparesis is a complex syndrome with symptoms that include nausea, vomiting, and postprandial abdominal pain, and is frequently accompanied by significant delays in gastric emptying. The pathophysiology of diabetic gastroparesis is fairly well understood; however, idiopathic gastroparesis, which accounts for one-third of all cases, may stem from infections, or autoimmune or neurologic disorders, among other causes. To date, few population-based studies have estimated the true prevalence and incidence of gastroparesis. Nonetheless, its prevalence appears to be rising, as does its incidence among minority populations, documented via hospitalizations, which can impose significant economic burdens on patients.

Gastroparesis can be divided into diabetic and nondiabetic, and the 3 main causes of gastroparesis are diabetic, postsurgical, and idiopathic. Delayed gastric emptying is the main manifestation of motility disorders for gastroparesis. Symptoms of gastroparesis are nonspecific and severity can vary. Nausea and vomiting are more common in diabetic gastroparesis whereas abdominal pain and early satiety are more frequent in idiopathic gastroparesis. Medication is still the mainstay of treatment of gastroparesis; however, the development of gastric electric stimulation and gastric peroral endoscopic pyloromyotomy brings more options for the treatment of diabetic and nondiabetic gastroparesis.

Although gastroparesis was described more than 60 years ago, the natural history and the long-term outcome are still being clarified. The patients with more severe gastroparesis often seek health care treatment in university medical centers specializing in gastrointestinal motility disorders and hence reports in the literature tend to be based on this population and may not be representative of the entire spectrum. The clinical manifestations of gastroparesis are heterogeneous but a significant proportion of patients end up with substantially poorer quality of life. In this article, the focus is on the clinical presentation and natural history of gastroparesis.

There is substantial overlap between the symptoms of gastroparesis and a variety of alternative disorders. These conditions include rumination syndrome, drug-induced gastric emptying delay, cannabinoid hyperemesis syndrome, and eating disorders, which can be identified based on the history alone. The remaining patients require a diagnostic approach of physical examination, laboratory tests, evaluation with esophagogastroduodenoscopy or contrast radiography, and a test to measure gastric emptying. Symptomatic patients who have normal nutritional status and gastric emptying that is either normal or mildly delayed should be diagnosed with functional dyspepsia, whereas patients with moderate or severe gastric emptying delay are diagnosed with gastroparesis.

Gastroparesis is a chronic and debilitating neuromuscular disorder of the upper gastrointestinal tract. Symptoms of gastroparesis include nausea, vomiting, epigastric pain, early satiety, and weight loss. Treating gastroparesis can be difficult. Dietary changes may improve symptoms in patients with mild disease. A variety of medications can be used to treat symptoms of nausea and vomiting, although most have not been subjected to randomized controlled trials and only one is approved by the Food and Drug Administration (metoclopramide). Pain management is essential, as nearly 90% of patients report symptoms of epigastric pain. This article reviews treatment options for symptoms of gastroparesis.

Patients with gastroparesis sometimes suffer from intractable nausea and vomiting, abdominal pain, and bloating, as well as a host of other symptoms that can often be difficult to control. Initially, patients are treated conservatively; some do well with conservative management but unfortunately some do not. Over the years, studies have shown the benefits of gastric electrical stimulation, which often results in symptomatic improvement and improvement in gastric emptying times. This article discusses the history of gastric electrical stimulation and its use in clinical practice to help those suffering from gastroparesis that is refractory to conservative medical management.

Gastroparesis is a debilitating chronic condition of indeterminate cause. Although conservative management is the mainstay of treatment, a significant percentage of patients will need interventions. Interventions range

from supportive measures, such as feeding tubes, to more radical surgeries, including endoscopic pyloromyotomy (per oral pyloromyotomy),
laparoscopic pyloroplasty, laparoscopic gastric stimulator placement,
and even subtotal or total gastrectomy. The authors present some current
treatment algorithms focused on the treatment side of the spectrum along
with outcomes data to support the various approaches.

Refractory gastroparesis is among the most difficult therapeutic challenges in gastroenterology. Pyloric dysfunction has been described in a
subset of patients with gastroparesis, prompting experimentation with
botulinum toxin injections into the pylorus, which is relatively safe and
has been successfully used in other gastrointestinal disorders. However,
causality between pyloric dysfunction and symptoms of gastroparesis
has never been demonstrated. Although several open-label studies
showed initial promise, 2 randomized clinical trials failed to elicit a difference in clinical outcomes in botulinum toxin versus placebo. Based on
current evidence, further use of botulinum toxin for gastroparesis is
discouraged outside of a research trial.

Gastroparesis is a syndrome of delayed gastric emptying. First-line treatment includes prokinetic medications. Those refractory to medical treatment are occasionally considered for endoscopic or surgical treatment
options, with unpredictable response. The pylorus plays a key role in
gastric emptying, with pylorospasm as the underlying mechanism of gastroparesis in some patients. Procedures aiming at disruption of the pylorus have improved gastroparesis symptoms in this subset of patients.
These include transpyloric stenting, used for inpatients with refractory
symptoms to allow hospital discharge or as a triage to assess symptoms
response in patients considered for more definite therapies such as
pyloromyotomy.

Gastric peroral endoscopic pyloromyotomy (G-POEM or POP) is a
feasible and effective procedure for the treatment of refractory gastroparesis. G-POEM is a technically demanding endoscopic procedure.
As of yet, there is no consensus on the technique. A variety of techniques have been reported in published studies. The essential technical
steps of the procedure are (1) establishment of submucosal tunnel in
gastric antrum, (2) identification of the pyloric muscular ring, (3) selective
circular myotomy, and (4) a 2.5-cm to 3.0-cm length of myotomy. There
are still some technical questions unanswered, and more studies are
needed to establish standardized techniques and possible improvement
of outcomes.

Gastric emptying scintigraphy (GES) helps to diagnose gastroparesis and is typically only used for whole stomach retention patterns. However, it may provide significantly more information when looking specifically at proximal and distal retention patterns. This article reviews global GES changes following gastric per oral endoscopic myotomy; how global, proximal, and distal GES measurements correlate to gastroparesis symptoms; and how proximal and distal GES may serve as proxies for the various mechanisms involved in gastroparesis. The authors' data on how GES may be used to select which patients will have success from G-POEM is also reviewed.

 Video content accompanies this article at http://www.giendo. theclinics.com/.

Gastroparesis is a challenging functional gastroenterological disorder, the complex pathophysiology of which hampers development of therapeutic modalities. Per-oral pyloromyotomy (POP) is a promising endoscopic therapy with a short-term clinical success rate of greater than 80%. Interest in POP is increasing, particularly in France, a country in which there is considerable expertise in submucosal endoscopy and functional disorders. Long-term follow-up and pyloric function evaluation are needed to assess the efficacy of POP in gastroparetic patients.

Per oral endoscopic pyloromyotomy (POP) has emerged as an endoscopic intervention for refractory gastroparesis. Early experience in the United States showed exciting clinical response rate, reduced gastroparesis symptoms, improved quality of life, and decreased gastric-emptying time during midterm follow-up up to 18 months. One recent study also showed that the number of patient emergency room visits and hospitalizations decreased significantly after POP. The procedure is technically feasible and safe. As more data become available, it is important to identify patients who would benefit most from this novel procedure.

GASTROINTESTINAL ENDOSCOPY CLINICS OF NORTH AMERICA

RELATED CLINICS SERIES

Gastroenterology Clinics
Clinics in Liver Disease

THE CLINICS ARE AVAILABLE ONLINE!
Access your subscription at:
www.theclinics.com

Foreword

Gastroparesis: New Approaches in Management

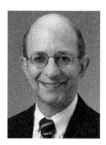

Charles J. Lightdale, MD
Consulting Editor

Gastroparesis is a chronic condition marked by the abnormally slow emptying of gastric contents into the duodenum. Symptoms include bloating, heartburn, and early satiety and can progress to nausea, vomiting, weight loss, and malnutrition. Diabetes is a major cause, as are autoimmune and collagen-vascular disorders and postsurgical states. While the cause of gastroparesis is often idiopathic, potentially reversible medication-related effects should always be considered. The condition is notoriously difficult to treat. New developments in management of gastroparesis, however, prompted me to devote this issue of *Gastrointestinal Endoscopy Clinics of North America* to this subject.

Dr Huimin Chen and Dr Qiang Cai, the editors for this issue, are to be congratulated for providing a comprehensive and current review of gastroparesis and assembling a remarkable international group of expert authors. Topical articles cover the epidemiology and pathophysiology of gastroparesis, a comparison of diabetic and non-diabetic-related patients, and detailed clinical manifestations. A key topic for clinicians covers the best modern methods for evaluation and diagnosis of patients with suspected gastroparesis.

Current treatment approaches to gastroparesis are the major feature of this issue. Symptomatic management, including dietary and pharmacologic treatments, is presented, as are surgical therapies. The use and potential benefits of implantable gastric electrical stimulation are covered in detail. Gastrointestinal endoscopists will be most interested in endoscopy-guided treatments, such as the use of botulinum toxin injections and placement of stents across the pyloric valve. Perhaps the most exciting new endoscopic treatment approach to gastroparesis has evolved from the success of per-oral endoscopic myotomy for esophageal achalasia: endoscopic pyloromyotomy (GPOEM), performed by the creation of an endoscopic submucosal tunnel extending through the gastric antrum to the pyloric muscle, which is then incised. Technical

Gastrointest Endoscopy Clin N Am 29 (2019) xiii–xiv
https://doi.org/10.1016/j.giec.2018.09.002
1052-5157/19/© 2018 Published by Elsevier Inc.

aspects are thoroughly described for GPOEM, and results are presented with outcomes and a look to the future for this novel endoscopic procedure. Altogether, this issue of *Gastrointestinal Endoscopy Clinics of North America* provides a terrific resource for gastroenterologists and interventional endoscopists in diagnosing and managing patients with gastroparesis.

Charles J. Lightdale, MD
Department of Medicine
Columbia University Medical Center
161 Fort Washington Avenue
New York, NY 10032, USA

E-mail address:
CJL18@columbia.edu

Preface

Gastroparesis: Current Opinions and New Endoscopic Therapies

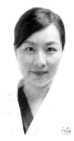 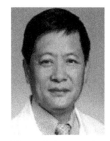

Huimin Chen, MD, PhD   Qiang Cai, MD, PhD
Editors

Gastroparesis is a disease with a complex pathophysiology that is not yet fully understood. Antroduodenal hypomotility, impaired fundic accommodation, and pylorospasm are believed to play major roles in delaying gastric emptying. Patients with gastroparesis suffer from frequent nausea, vomiting, earlier satiety, regurgitation, and so forth. Diabetes is the most common cause. Other causes include gastrointestinal surgery, some disorders of the nervous system, such as Parkinson disease and stroke, and some medicines, such as tricyclic antidepressants, calcium channel blockers, and opiate pain relievers and others. Common therapies, such as dietary modification and medications, are usually not very effective. Interventional therapies, such as gastric electrical stimulation, botulinum injection, pylorus stenting, and surgical pyloromyotomy, also have limited effect. Patients with gastroparesis usually end up with frequent emergency room visits and hospitalization.

In this issue of *Gastrointestinal Endoscopy Clinics of North America*, a group of world experts on gastroparesis have updated the current knowledge of gastroparesis from the pathophysiology and clinical manifestations to new therapies.

The physiology of gastric motility involves orchestrated interactions between each area of the stomach in a cellular level, an example of which was demonstrated by a stimulation of antroduodenal phasic motor activity by mechanically distending the gastric fundus. Therefore, a mechanical disruption of the pyloric muscle may have effects beyond local pyloric dilation, but also on global gastric emptying as well. This theory was demonstrated by recent studies on surgical pyloroplasty that improved both symptoms score and gastric emptying time. However, it is reasonable to hypothesize that pylorus-directed therapy such as pyloric stenting, intrapyloric botulinum injection, and gastric per oral endoscopic pyloromyotomy (GPOEM or POP) would be most effective in patients whose symptoms manifest from pyloric dysfunction. The challenging part is to identify those patients who would most benefit from this novel

Gastrointest Endoscopy Clin N Am 29 (2019) xv–xvi
https://doi.org/10.1016/j.giec.2018.09.001
1052-5157/19/© 2018 Published by Elsevier Inc.

procedure. Some studies have already shown a promising short-term outcome of GPOEM, but the long-term outcome of GPOEM is unknown.

Gastroparesis affects approximately 5 to 10 million adult Americans. The persistent symptoms of pain, nausea, and vomiting reduce patients' quality of life and impose a significant negative economic impact on the health care system. It is difficult to treat and also difficult to predict responses to therapy. No biomarkers have been identified that predict therapeutic response, and medications designed to accelerate gastric emptying may not lead to symptom improvement. A validated treatment algorithm does not exist at the present time, and head-to-head studies comparing different therapeutic modalities and innovative solutions, including new medications and new interventional therapies, are needed to establish better care for patients with gastroparesis.

Huimin Chen, MD, PhD
Division of Gastroenterology and Hepatology
Renji Hospital, School of Medicine
Shanghai Jiao Tong University
Shanghai 200127, China

Qiang Cai, MD, PhD
Division of Digestive Diseases
Emory University School of Medicine
Atlanta 30322, GA, USA

E-mail addresses:
huimin.chan@foxmail.com (H. Chen)
qcai@emory.edu (Q. Cai)

Epidemiology and Pathophysiology of Gastroparesis

Baha Moshiree, MD, MS-CI[a,b,]*, Michael Potter, MD[c,d],
Nicholas J. Talley, MD, PhD[e]

KEYWORDS

- Gastroparesis • Functional dyspepsia • Epidemiology • Prevalence • Incidence
- Risk factors • Quality of life

KEY POINTS

- Gastroparesis, although seemingly still rare, poses a significant burden to society and exhausts health care resources with frequent hospitalizations and work absenteeism.
- Although the pathophysiology of gastroparesis is now better understood, idiopathic gastroparesis remains the most common subgroup, with an expanding number of etiologies that are now better understood.
- The prevalence of gastroparesis is rising, especially among children and minority groups, possibly due to a rise in diabetes around the world.
- A diagnosis of gastroparesis is associated with increased morbidity and decreased survival, especially in the elderly, as compared with unspecified dyspepsia or nausea and vomiting from other causes.

INTRODUCTION

Gastroparesis is a challenging disorder for both patients and clinicians. Given its increasing prevalence, incidence, and hospitalization rates, gastroparesis is becoming increasingly burdensome to health care systems, and the significant morbidity associated with the disorder can significantly impact patients' quality of life, leading to frequent work absenteeism, thus posing a further socioeconomic burden.[1,2] The underlying

Disclosure Statement: Medtronic (Given Imaging), Cairn Diagnostics and Allergan (B. Moshiree). Nothing to disclose (M. Potter, N.J Talley).
[a] Division of Gastroenterology, University of North Carolina, 1025 Morehead Medical Drive Suite 300, Charlotte, NC 28204, USA; [b] Atrium Health, Carolinas HealthCare System, Digestive Health-Morehead Medical Plaza, 1025 Morehead Medical Drive, Suite 300, Charlotte, NC 28204, USA; [c] Department of Gastroenterology, University of Newcastle, HMRI Building, Kookaburra Circuit, New Lambton Heights, New South Wales 2305, Australia; [d] Department of Gastroenterology, John Hunter Hospital, Lookout Road, New Lambton Heights, New South Wales 2305, Australia; [e] Global Research, Digestive and Health Neurogastroenterology, New Lambton, NSW 2305, Australia
* Corresponding author.
E-mail address: baha.moshiree@atriumhealth.org

pathogenesis of the disorder is not well understood, but recent research has begun to shine some light on the mechanisms underlying gastroparesis, especially diabetic gastroparesis. This review focuses on the epidemiology and pathophysiology of gastroparesis.

DEFINITIONS

Gastroparesis is a clinical syndrome defined by symptoms and delayed gastric emptying in the absence of a mechanical obstruction; characteristic symptoms are considered to include early satiety, nausea, vomiting, postprandial fullness, and epigastric or abdominal pain.[3,4] Symptoms of gastroparesis have considerable overlap with those of functional dyspepsia, which is defined by the Rome IV criteria (**Table 1**). Symptoms of functional dyspepsia also include early satiety and postprandial fullness (functional dyspepsia postprandial distress subtype), as well as epigastric pain and epigastric burning (functional dyspepsia epigastric pain subtype), but not predominantly nausea with vomiting or weight loss as often seen with gastroparesis.[5,6] Symptoms of both gastroparesis and functional dyspepsia are chronic, occurring at least weekly for a minimum of 6 months in functional dyspepsia according to the Rome IV criteria[5] and for more than 3 months for gastroparesis by consensus, although the time frames are arbitrary.[7]

Controversy exits over whether gastroparesis and functional dyspepsia are related disorders or whether gastroparesis is a subset of functional dyspepsia; as both may arise postinfection and manifest very similar symptoms, the distinction may be arbitrary and unhelpful.[8,9] This overlap in symptoms can lead to misdiagnosis in clinical practice, although data on the prevalence and impact of misdiagnosis are lacking.[10] Up to one-third of patients with functional dyspepsia will demonstrate delayed gastric emptying, whereas fewer than 5% will have rapid gastric emptying.[11,12] Duodenal micro-inflammation, characterized by increased duodenal eosinophilia, has been observed in functional dyspepsia but has not been studied in idiopathic gastroparesis.[13,14] Taken together, the observations suggest that these 2 conditions may lie at the ends of a pathophysiologic spectrum with severe delay in gastric emptying at one end in gastroparesis (defined as 4-hour % gastric retention of >30%) and normal or only a modest delay (or uncommonly even rapid emptying) at the other end with functional dyspepsia.[10]

Table 1
Differentiating functional dyspepsia and gastroparesis

Findings	Gastroparesis	Functional Dyspepsia
Pathophysiology	Motility and sensory dysfunction Interstitial cells of Cajal loss	Sensory dysfunction Impaired accommodation
Predominant symptoms	Nausea, vomiting, and postprandial pain predominate Weight loss often occurs	Early satiation, postprandial fullness, epigastric pain or burning
Diagnosis	Gastric scintigraphy, wireless motility capsule, C^{13} Spirulina breath testing	Rome IV criteria
Gastric scintigraphy findings: Delay, rapid, normal	Delayed	1/3 delayed, <5% rapid, 2/3 normal
Symptom duration	Acute or >3 mo Waxing and waning	Symptom onset 6 mo, duration 3 mo with symptoms occurring 3 d/wk
Proton pump inhibitor use	May delay gastric emptying	Helps symptoms
Tricyclic antidepressants	+/− benefit	Benefit symptoms

ETIOLOGY OF GASTROPARESIS

The etiology of gastroparesis varies widely, with more than 90 causes identified, but most studies have observed that between 30% and 50% of patients have an unidentified cause, referred to as "idiopathic" gastroparesis.[15] Other common causes of gastroparesis include systemic and metabolic disorders, with the most common reported being diabetes mellitus (25%), drugs (22%), postsurgical causes (7%), and others, such as Parkinson disease, connective tissue diseases, and known infections such as enteroviruses.[16-18]

By some estimates, as many as 25% to 55% of patients with type 1 diabetes have gastroparesis, with a slightly higher incidence rate in patients with type 2 diabetes, although other studies less prone to selection bias have documented a much lower incidence rate of 5% of patients with type 1 diabetes developing symptoms of gastroparesis over a 10-year period.[19] Once patients experience symptoms of diabetic gastroparesis, the syndrome usually persists, regardless of improvements in glycemic control.[3,20] This persistence of diabetic gastroparesis probably stems from patients with both type 1 and type 2 diabetes having smooth muscle abnormalities, with a loss of the interstitial cells of Cajal (ICC) impairing gastric motor coordination and leading to delayed emptying,[17-19] as well as decreases in protective macrophages in the antrum.[21,22]

Medications may contribute to cases of "idiopathic" gastroparesis, yet be underrecognized. Proton pump inhibitors (PPIs), used commonly to treat gastroesophageal reflux disease (GERD) and the epigastric burning that can accompany gastroparesis and functional dyspepsia, may impair intragastric peptic digestion and thus delay gastric emptying of solids.[23] PPIs are often administered in those with suspected refractory GERD, but some of these patients may in fact have unrecognized underlying gastroparesis inducing reflux.[3] A systematic review of 25 studies focusing on the impact of PPIs on gastric emptying returned mixed results. Only 5 studies documented significant delay in gastric emptying from omeprazole or rabeprazole.[20] Three of these 5 studies used both a solid meal to assess gastric transit times and reliable methods (scintigraphy or a breath test) to document significant delays in solid but not liquid gastric emptying. In contrast to PPIs, tricyclic antidepressants, which are effective in treating the visceral hypersensitivity in functional dyspepsia, do not delay gastric emptying despite being anticholinergic and are therefore not contraindicated for treatment of gastroparesis,[24] although a multicenter trial using nortriptyline found it not superior to placebo for treatment of gastroparesis.[25,26] Glucagonlike peptide (GLP)-1 agonists are commonly used to treat type 2 diabetes, but GLP-1 agonists are known to slow gastric motility, reduce food intake, and increase satiety, and should be of limited use in patients with known diabetic gastroparesis.[27] Narcotics should be discontinued, as they often exacerbate gastroparesis symptoms. The cannabinoid CB1 receptor agonists inhibit acetylcholine release and can therefore slow gastric emptying in humans, despite the antiemetic effect of its tetrahydrocannabinol component.[15,24,28]

Gastroparesis can be precipitated by surgical procedures, including Nissen fundoplication, bariatric surgery, cholecystectomy, and other gastric bypass procedures, such as Roux-en-Y gastrojejunostomy.[29] Although vagus nerve damage is suspected if symptoms are chronic, many cases resolve within a year of fundoplication.[30] Patients with biliary dyskinesia often have upper gastrointestinal symptoms similar to those with gastroparesis; some studies have shown a prevalence of idiopathic gastroparesis in as high as 45% of those who underwent cholecystectomy, with one-third of patients having biliary dyskinesia as the only reason for surgery.[31] The National Institute of Diabetes and Digestive and Kidney Diseases (NIDDK) Gastroparesis Clinical Research Consortium has reported a history of prior cholecystectomy in 36% of their

391 patients recruited, many of whom had several other comorbidities, such as fibromyalgia, anxiety, and depression.[32] Although this finding does not imply causation, it suggests that patients with gastroparesis and prior history of cholecystectomy have a worse quality of life than those without prior surgery.

Neurologic diseases can also cause gastroparesis, with Parkinson disease the most often implicated.[33] Patients with Parkinson disease frequently report nausea, early satiety, and bloating, with several studies using gastric emptying scintigraphy or breath testing confirming the presence of gastroparesis.[34,35] Studies have also demonstrated that delayed gastric emptying can lengthen times to plasma levodopa peak in patients with Parkinson disease, as orally administered levodopa delays jejunal absorption, limiting the efficacy of the medication and worsening gastroparesis.[35] Studies have also reported gastroparesis in patients with multiple sclerosis, which may both deplete the ICCs and damage the enteric nervous system.[36]

Small-duct pancreatitis is a risk factor for gastroparesis, with significantly delayed gastric emptying seen in 44% of patients, perhaps related to the effect of high cholecystokinin levels present as a result of pancreatic hyperstimulation.[37] In these patients, gastroparesis may interfere with pancreatic enzyme therapy by limiting the absorption of exogenous pancreatic supplementation to the duodenum. Patients with cystic fibrosis are also at risk of developing gastroparesis. A systematic review by Corral and colleagues[38] identified gastroparesis in 38% (95% confidence interval [CI] 30%–45%) of 359 patients with cystic fibrosis, although the diagnostic modality for diagnosis of slow gastric emptying was varied in the 19 pooled studies.

Connective tissue diseases have also been linked with gastroparesis, including scleroderma, systemic lupus, and mixed connective tissue disease.[17,39] Patients with scleroderma or lupus have gastroparesis probably due to smooth muscle atrophy and myopathy.[40] Notably, Ehlers-Danlos syndrome may account for some of the idiopathic cases of gastroparesis, with up to one-third of patients seeking treatment for gastroparesis having undiagnosed joint hypermobility.[16] This is especially prevalent in the hypermobility subtype of Ehlers-Danlos, type III, which has no known genetic basis.[41]

Finally, viral infections are potential causes of idiopathic gastroparesis, with the natural history often characterized by an acute onset following a prodrome or viral infection, with symptoms remaining for months or even years before spontaneously resolving.[18,42] Gastric enterovirus infections have been found by immunostaining of gastric antral and fundic biopsies in patients with idiopathic gastroparesis, many of whom had malnutrition.[43] In pediatric patients, neuroenteric staining of the myenteric plexus has identified loss of ICCs, evidence of inflammation in proximity to neuronal bodies, other degenerative changes in the ganglion cells, and neuronal hypertrophy, supporting a possible infectious cause of gastroparesis[43] (**Figs. 1** and **2A, B**).

EPIDEMIOLOGY OF GASTROPARESIS
Prevalence of Gastroparesis

Well-conducted studies regarding the prevalence of gastroparesis, using both the presence of symptoms along with demonstrable delayed gastric emptying diagnosed by gastric emptying scintigraphy are lacking. Only one population-based study from Olmsted County, Minnesota, has addressed the prevalence of gastroparesis using these criteria.[17] Jung and colleagues[17] used a medical record linkage system to identify community residents with gastroparesis based on strict definitions including the presence of typical symptoms of up to 3 months, and documented delayed gastric emptying on either endoscopy or upper gastrointestinal endoscopy. They identified 83 patients who had definite diagnosis of gastroparesis based on these criteria, and

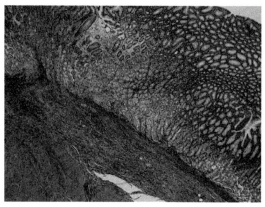

Fig. 1. Trichrome stain showing fibrosis in the submucosa and muscularis of the stomach in a patient with gastroparesis (original magnification ×40). (*Courtesy of* Shamaila Waseem MD, Carmel, IN.)

a further 44 with probable gastroparesis. They reported a prevalence of definite gastroparesis per 100,000 persons of 37.8 in women (95% CI 23.3–52.4) versus 9.6 in men (95% CI 1.8–17.4). This study was conducted in a predominantly White community, and data regarding the prevalence of gastroparesis in Hispanic or black populations are lacking. Hospital discharge information, such as the study by Wadhwa and colleagues,[44] suggests that the prevalence of gastroparesis in minority populations may be increasing. Their retrospective analysis of the largest US inpatient database documents hospital discharges, provides a picture of large population trends over time, albeit limited by ICD-9 codes and hospitalizations only; they reported increases in the prevalence of gastroparesis as a diagnosis in black and Hispanic individuals over white individuals, in terms of increases in hospital discharges, over a 16-year period. During this time, black patients with gastroparesis had hospital discharges increase 4.5-fold, Hispanic patients, 5.5-fold, and white patients, 3.0-fold.[44]

Diabetic Gastroparesis

The prevalence of diabetic gastroparesis in tertiary referral centers is reported to be 30% to 50% of type 1 diabetes and 15% to 30% of type 2 diabetes[45,46]; however, selection bias and lack of strict diagnostic criteria have likely overestimated the true prevalence in these populations.

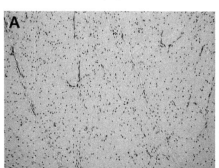
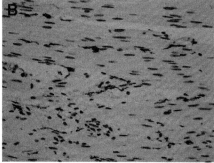

Fig. 2. (*A*) CD 117 immunostaining showing absence of ICCs in muscularis propria. (*B*) CD 117 immunostain showing normal number and distribution of ICCs. (*Courtesy of* Shamaila Waseem MD, Carmel, IN.)

The only population-based study of diabetic gastroparesis using strict diagnostic criteria was based in Olmsted County, Minnesota, which used the database from the Rochester Epidemiology Study medical records database.[17] Choung and colleagues[19] followed a cohort of type 1 and type 2 diabetic individuals over an 11-year period, and calculated the cumulative prevalence of gastroparesis (based on delayed gastric emptying scintigraphy and typical symptoms); the cumulative risk of developing gastroparesis was 5.2% of patients with type 1 diabetes, and 1.1% among those with type 2 diabetes. The presence of heartburn at baseline was significantly associated with the risk of gastroparesis (hazard ratio 6.6, 95% CI 1.7–25).[19]

Incidence (New Onset) of Gastroparesis

Again, the Rochester Epidemiology Study allowed for the only well-designed study addressing the incidence of gastroparesis in the community. The Mayo clinic's medical records system collects data on 80% of the population, with 96% being seen within a 4-year period, allowing for accurate estimation of incidence.[17] Using these data, and a strict definition of gastroparesis based on delayed gastric emptying and typical symptoms, Jung and colleagues[17] reported an incidence rate for gastroparesis per 100,000 person years of 9.8 for women and 2.4 for men. The rate was higher in older people, with an incidence rate of 10.5 in patients aged 60 years and older.

RISK FACTORS AND PREDICTORS OF PROGRESSION
Influence of Age and Gender

Numerous studies have found significantly higher risks for gastroparesis associated with gender and age. In particular, studies have identified women in most cases of gastroparesis, with women nearly 4 times likelier to be diagnosed with gastroparesis than men[17,47] (Table 2). The increased risk may be due in part to higher health care–seeking behavior in women,[44] but underlying pathophysiological differences may also play a key role, including increased progesterone levels[48] or possibly increased immune activation in women. Hormonal regulation may contribute to the gender differences seen in gastroparesis, specifically the role played by progesterone. During the follicular and luteal phases of the menstrual cycle, rises in progesterone levels significantly impact gastric emptying. Progesterone acts as a relaxant on the smooth muscle in the gut, promoting hypomotility and delaying gastric emptying. Moreover, progesterone upregulates symptoms of gastroparesis significantly during both pregnancy and the luteal phases of menstrual cycles.[48] Similarly, increased age is associated with gastroparesis, with increasing incidence seen in older age groups, which may reflect more time for exposure to infectious agents, drugs, or other unknown factors.[17,49]

Glycemic Control and Diabetic Gastroparesis

Both type 1 and type 2 diabetes and poor glycemic control account for both increased risk of gastroparesis and progression in the severity of symptoms.[50] Elevated blood glucose concentrations (>8 mmol/L) are associated with delayed gastric emptying.[46]

Small Intestinal Bacterial Overgrowth

Whether small intestinal bacterial overgrowth (SIBO) is a risk factor for gastroparesis or a comorbid condition is a matter of debate. However, in patients with small bowel dysmotility, SIBO often develops; loss of the ICCs induces decreased migrating motor complexes responsible for adequate movement of undigested contents, promoting a change in the gut microbiota.[51] In a retrospective study of more than 990 patients with upper gastrointestinal symptoms using D-xylose breath testing, slightly more than half

Table 2
Demographic of patients with gastroparesis by the International Foundation for Functional Gastrointestinal Disorders gastroparesis survey over 9.3 years (survey results of North America including Canada and Mexico, based on 1423 subjects)

Demographics	Data in Mean ± SD (Median, Range) or Frequency (%)
Age at time of questionnaire, y	44.2 ± 13.9 (44, 18–89)
Age at start of symptoms, y	34.9 ± 16.0 (35, 1–82)
Age at diagnosis, y	39.9 ± 14.0 (40, 4–82)
Years between start of symptoms and diagnosis	5.0 ± 8.5 (2, 0–64)
Duration of symptoms, y	9.3 ± 10.0 (6, 0–73)
Body mass index	26.7 ± 8.0 (25.0, 12.1–66.3)
Female gender	1321 (92.8)
Race/ethnicity	
White or other non-Hispanic	1235 (86.8)
Black or African American	45 (3.2)
Hispanic, Latino, or Spanish	64 (4.5)
American Indian, Asian, Pacific Islander	25 (1.7)
Other	54 (3.8)
Location	
United States	1251 (87.9)
Canada	47 (3.3)
Mexico	2 (0.1)
Other	123 (8.6)

From Yu D, Ramsey FV, Norton WF, et al. The burdens, concerns, and quality of life of patients with gastroparesis. Dig Dis Sci 2017;62:882; with permission.

of the patients tested positive for SIBO, with a significant association among SIBO, gastroesophageal reflux disease, and gastroparesis.[52] In addition, patients with gastroparesis had a later peak in the rise of methane hydrogen at 120 minutes compared with the patients with SIBO and normal gastric emptying scintigraphy.

Pathophysiology of Gastroparesis

The pathophysiology of gastroparesis is not well understood, but of the various causes of gastroparesis, diabetes is the best understood. In diabetic gastroparesis, potential mechanisms include denervation of the vagus nerve, loss of nitric oxide synthase in enteric nerves, loss of the ICCs, and lack of expression neuronal nitric oxide.[23,53] New insights suggest a disruption of the ICC networks regulating gastrointestinal motility and a paucity of nerve bodies. The decrease in the ICCs found in patients with diabetic (and some cases of idiopathic) gastroparesis may cause the delayed emptying, which impairs motor coordination.[54] A histologic study on transmural gastric corpus specimens in patients with diabetic and idiopathic gastroparesis, and controls found a significant decrease in the number of ICCs in both diabetic and idiopathic gastroparesis patients compared with controls.[55] Moreover, a significant correlation has been found between the number of CD206+ macrophages and depletion of the ICCs in patients with diabetic gastroparesis and diabetic controls, suggesting that in humans, CD206+ macrophages may play a protective role in preserving ICCs, a finding that may guide the development of novel targeted treatment options[22] (**Fig. 3**A–C). The findings are consistent with earlier studies in animal models of type 1 diabetes, in which loss of CD206+ heme oxygenase-1 (HO-1) expressing M2 macrophages was found to increase the oxidative stress and loss of ICC function, which led to delayed gastric emptying and gastroparesis.[56] This delay can theoretically be reversed by induction of HO-1 with hemin, but clinical studies have failed to confirm the hypothesis.[57] Furthermore, response to gastric electrical stimulation with the Enterra device (Medtronic, Fridley, MN) has been seen in those patients with normal numbers of ICCs in patients with refractory gastroparesis (34 diabetic individuals, 5 idiopathic, 2 postsurgical).[58]

Less is known about the pathophysiology of idiopathic gastroparesis aside from loss of the ICCs, as seen also in diabetic gastroparesis. Upper gastrointestinal symptoms in gastroparesis may result from a variety of mechanisms, including impaired gastric accommodation, hypomotility of the gastric antrum, and visceral hyperalgesia.[3] Some patients with idiopathic gastroparesis may have elevated pyloric pressures and thus severely delayed gastric emptying due to decreased distensibility of the pylorus, which leads to nausea and vomiting.[59] In EndoFLIP, the functional lumen imaging probe (FLIP) assesses pyloric sphincter function by measuring pyloric pressure and distensibility. In one study of EndoFLIP, pyloric diameter and cross-sectional area were negatively correlated with postprandial fullness and early satiety, suggesting pyloric stenosis plays a role in these symptoms of gastroparesis.[60] In the future, this may predict response to pyloric botulinum toxin injection, dilatation, or pyloromyotomy, all often empirically performed in patients with gastroparesis but that have not been proven to lead to improved gastric emptying in randomized trials.[61]

Impact of Gastroparesis on Health-Related Quality of Life

Most studies of the impact of gastroparesis on patients' quality of life rely on the well-validated Patient Assessment of Upper Gastrointestinal Disorders-Quality of Life (PAGI-QOL).[62] Nevertheless, even this tool may fail to correctly capture patients' quality of life accurately in the presence of a syndrome with a severity that consistently waxes and wanes throughout the day and night.[63] Pain, nausea, postprandial fullness, and early satiety in gastroparesis often lead to poor eating and malnutrition stemming from a calorie-deficient diet and inadequate absorption of vitamins and minerals.[3] In patients who have gastroparesis with Parkinson disease as the underlying etiology, gastroparesis may exacerbate weight loss, in addition to impacting the absorption of dopamine agonists, which can lead to a worsening of neurologic symptoms.[64]

A study by Parkman and colleagues[65] of patients with diabetic and idiopathic gastroparesis reported lower scores on quality of life measures and higher rates of

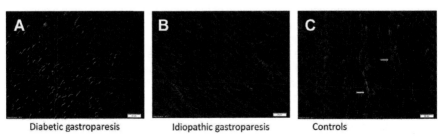

Diabetic gastroparesis   Idiopathic gastroparesis   Controls

Fig. 3. Depicting stomach biopsies in patients with diabetic (A) and idiopathic gastroparesis (B) having loss of ICCs by immunofluorescence staining (see *arrows*) as compared with controls (C). (*Courtesy of* Madhusudan Grover MD, Rochester, MN.)

comorbidities in patients with diabetic gastroparesis than in those with idiopathic gastroparesis. However, this study population came from the NIDDK Gastroparesis Registry, where patients were likelier to be women, white, and educated and therefore perhaps are not representative of the US population with gastroparesis at large.

Gastroparesis has other significant impacts on patients' quality of life, including persistent pain, rated as severe in 70% of patients in a study by Hasler and colleagues[66] of 393 patients who demonstrated delayed gastric emptying on gastric emptying scintigraphy. In the same study, pain was significantly associated with the greatest impact on quality of life, with many patients also reporting depression and anxiety. Likewise, a study by Cherian and colleagues[67] of patients with gastroparesis found that pain interfered with sleep in 66% of patients and eating in 72%, which further impacted patients' quality of life. Depression is reported in 23% of patients with idiopathic gastroparesis, and may reflect not only the disruptions created by chronic pain on daily living but also the challenges faced by patients for whom treatments for gastroparesis have only limited effectiveness.[3,15] Other larger studies using the International Foundation for Functional Gastrointestinal disorders survey questionnaire in 1423 adults patients in North America with symptom duration of 9.3 years have found that most patients with gastroparesis are dissatisfied with treatments (33%), and in particular patients younger than 45 years, women, and those of white race reported a significantly decreased quality of life as assessed by the SF-36, which negatively correlated with symptoms of nausea ($r = -0.37$), upper abdominal pain ($r = -0.37$), and early satiety ($r = -0.37$).[47]

Hospitalizations and Economic Burden of Gastroparesis

A major impact of gastroparesis that is relatively underreported in the literature is the economic burden that stems not only from clinic visits, hospitalizations, and treatments, but also from underemployment or unemployment. In a study of 55 patients, Bielefeldt and colleagues[68] reported that, despite a mean age younger than 45 years, only one-quarter of the study population was employed, and more than half had incomes significantly below the national average. A further subset of study patients with gastroparesis reported they had retired, gone on to a disability support pension, quit jobs, or halted their further education due to symptoms of gastroparesis. The numbers of patients with gastroparesis who are unable to work or are on disability support pension may be higher than the far more widely recognized impacts of Crohn disease on the employment status of patients.[69]

Children with gastroparesis have been increasingly hospitalized for gastroparesis with costs 5.8-fold higher in 2013 as compared with 2004.[70] Although costs per hospitalization have not changed, the number of hospitalizations in the United States each year have risen from 252 per year to 1310.[70] This translates to a rate of increase in total annual cost of hospitalization for gastroparesis of approximately $3.4 million a year from 2004 to 2013 ($P = .0001$) (Fig. 4A, B). In adult patients with gastroparesis, the costs of hospitalizations have increased fourfold between 1997 and 2013. In addition, the costs of hospitalization for gastroparesis soared 159% between those 2 timepoints, despite the mean length of stays decreasing by 20%. With these rising costs, the aggregate charges for treating gastroparesis rose by a staggering 1026% during the same period.[70] These statistics mirror the trends identified by Wang and colleagues[49] between 1995 and 2004, when the mean length of stay for hospitalization for gastroparesis decreased by more than half a day, whereas the costs of hospitalization more than doubled.

Diabetic gastroparesis may have the most severe impact on patients, associated with more clinical visits and hospitalizations, as well as increased morbidity and mortality.[1]

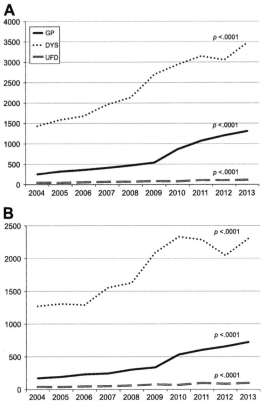

Fig. 4. (*A*) Number of hospitalizations each year for gastroparesis (GP), dyspepsia (DYS), and unspecified functional disorder of stomach (UFD) over time. (*B*) Total cost of hospitalizations for GP over time (millions USD). (*Adapted from* Lu PL, Moore-Clingenpeel M, Yacob D, et al. The rising cost of hospital care for children with gastroparesis: 2004-2013. Neurogastroenterol Motil 2016;28(11):1698–704; with permission.)

Hyett and colleagues[1] found that diabetic patients with gastroparesis established via standardized scintigraphy had significantly higher rates of hospitalization, and clinic and emergency room visits than diabetic patients without gastric delay on scintigraphy.

Morbidity and Mortality

Data on morbidity and mortality from gastroparesis are both mixed and limited, due to either the size of the population studied or the duration of the study. The 5-year study of 86 patients with gastroparesis by Kong and colleagues[71] showed no significant relationship between gastroparesis in patients diagnosed via gastric emptying scintigraphy and death. Hyett and colleagues[1] compared diabetic patients with gastroparesis diagnosed by gastric emptying scintigraphy, diabetic patients with symptoms of gastroparesis but normal gastric emptying, and diabetic patients without symptoms; there were no differences in mortality associated with having symptoms of gastroparesis or with higher hemoglobin A1c levels. Nevertheless, patients with delayed gastric emptying also had 12.8% higher rates for cardiovascular disease, which was a significant increase from those without delayed gastric emptying.[1] The 2009 study by Jung and colleagues[17] of the largely white population in Olmsted County, Minnesota, remains not only one of the lone, large, population-based studies on incidence and prevalence of gastroparesis, but also showed the impact from gastroparesis on mortality, with comparable diminishment of survival during a 5-year median follow-up of patients with symptoms of gastroparesis both with and without delayed gastric emptying. In contrast to the population without any symptoms of gastroparesis, who had an 81% 10-year survival rate, patients with any symptoms of gastroparesis had a survival rate of only 67% over 10 years (95% CI 60%–75%, $P<.01$). Older age at diagnosis was associated with worse survival. Unsurprisingly, patients with nondiabetic gastroparesis had a better survival rate than patients with diabetic gastroparesis, whereas idiopathic gastroparesis was associated with greater survival rates than nonidiopathic gastroparesis.[17]

SUMMARY

Gastroparesis is a complex syndrome characterized by severe upper gastrointestinal symptoms combined with delayed gastric emptying. Given the difficulties in identifying all cases in the community, the true prevalence and incidence of gastroparesis remain poorly understood. Regardless, it is seemingly a rare disorder, and most cases are either idiopathic or secondary to diabetes. Whereas the pathophysiology of diabetic gastroparesis is now better understood, idiopathic gastroparesis remains less well defined, and it is likely that unidentified factors, including infections, connective tissue diseases, neurologic syndromes, and autoimmune-related diseases contribute to this group. Gastroparesis is probably associated with an increased mortality, and the prevalence is rising, thereby posing a considerable personal and socioeconomic burden that needs to be better addressed.

REFERENCES

1. Hyett B, Martinez FJ, Gill BM, et al. Delayed radionucleotide gastric emptying studies predict morbidity in diabetics with symptoms of gastroparesis. Gastroenterology 2009;137:445–52.
2. Camilleri M, Dubois D, Coulie B, et al. Prevalence and socioeconomic impact of upper gastrointestinal disorders in the United States: results of the US upper gastrointestinal study. Clin Gastroenterol Hepatol 2005;3:543–52.
3. Camilleri M, Parkman HP, Shafi MA, et al. Clinical guideline: management of gastroparesis. Am J Gastroenterol 2013;108:18–37 [quiz: 38].
4. Moshiree B, Bollipo S, Horowitz M, et al. Epidemiology of gastroparesis. In: Parkman HP, McCallum RW, et al, editors. Gastroparesis: pathophysiology, presentation and treatment. New York: Springer Science & Business Media; 2011.
5. Stanghellini V, Chan FK, Hasler WL, et al. Gastroduodenal disorders. Gastroenterology 2016;150:1380–92.
6. Talley NJ, Ford AC. Functional dyspepsia. N Engl J Med 2015;373:1853–63.
7. Horowitz M, Su YC, Rayner CK, et al. Gastroparesis: prevalence, clinical significance and treatment. Can J Gastroenterol 2001;15:805–13.
8. Stanghellini V, Tosetti C, Paternico A, et al. Risk indicators of delayed gastric emptying of solids in patients with functional dyspepsia. Gastroenterology 1996;110:1036–42.
9. Talley NJ, Locke GR 3rd, Lahr BD, et al. Functional dyspepsia, delayed gastric emptying, and impaired quality of life. Gut 2006;55:933–9.
10. Pasricha PJ, Colvin R, Yates K, et al. Characteristics of patients with chronic unexplained nausea and vomiting and normal gastric emptying. Clin Gastroenterol Hepatol 2011;9:567–76.e1-4.
11. Stanghellini V, Tack J. Gastroparesis: separate entity or just a part of dyspepsia? Gut 2014;63:1972–8.

12. Tack J, Piessevaux H, Coulie B, et al. Role of impaired gastric accommodation to a meal in functional dyspepsia. Gastroenterology 1998;115:1346–52.
13. Talley NJ, Walker MM, Aro P, et al. Non-ulcer dyspepsia and duodenal eosinophilia: an adult endoscopic population-based case-control study. Clin Gastroenterol Hepatol 2007;5:1175–83.
14. Vanheel H, Vicario M, Boesmans W, et al. Activation of eosinophils and mast cells in functional dyspepsia: an ultrastructural evaluation. Sci Rep 2018;8:5383.
15. Soykan I, Sivri B, Sarosiek I, et al. Demography, clinical characteristics, psychological and abuse profiles, treatment, and long-term follow-up of patients with gastroparesis. Dig Dis Sci 1998;43:2398–404.
16. Fikree A, Grahame R, Aktar R, et al. A prospective evaluation of undiagnosed joint hypermobility syndrome in patients with gastrointestinal symptoms. Clin Gastroenterol Hepatol 2014;12:1680–7.e2.
17. Jung HK, Choung RS, Locke GR 3rd, et al. The incidence, prevalence, and outcomes of patients with gastroparesis in Olmsted County, Minnesota, from 1996 to 2006. Gastroenterology 2009;136:1225–33.
18. Barkin JA, Czul F, Barkin JS, et al. Gastric enterovirus infection: a possible causative etiology of gastroparesis. Dig Dis Sci 2016;61:2344–50.
19. Choung RS, Locke GR 3rd, Schleck CD, et al. Risk of gastroparesis in subjects with type 1 and 2 diabetes in the general population. Am J Gastroenterol 2012; 107:82–8.
20. Farrugia G. Histologic changes in diabetic gastroparesis. Gastroenterol Clin North Am 2015;44:31–8.
21. He CL, Soffer EE, Ferris CD, et al. Loss of interstitial cells of Cajal and inhibitory innervation in insulin-dependent diabetes. Gastroenterology 2001;121:427–34.
22. Grover M, Bernard CE, Pasricha PJ, et al. Diabetic and idiopathic gastroparesis is associated with loss of CD206-positive macrophages in the gastric antrum. Neurogastroenterol Motil 2017;29(6). https://doi.org/10.1111/nmo.13018.
23. Sanaka M, Yamamoto T, Kuyama Y. Effects of proton pump inhibitors on gastric emptying: a systematic review. Dig Dis Sci 2010;55:2431–40.
24. Talley NJ, Locke GR, Saito YA, et al. Effect of amitriptyline and escitalopram on functional dyspepsia: a multicenter, randomized controlled study. Gastroenterology 2015;149:340–9.e2.
25. Lacy BE, Saito YA, Camilleri M, et al. Effects of antidepressants on gastric function in patients with functional dyspepsia. Am J Gastroenterol 2018;113(2): 216–24.
26. Parkman HP, Van Natta ML, Abell TL, et al. Effect of nortriptyline on symptoms of idiopathic gastroparesis: the NORIG randomized clinical trial. JAMA 2013; 310(24):2640–9.
27. Derosa G, Maffioli P. GLP-1 agonists exenatide and liraglutide: a review about their safety and efficacy. Curr Clin Pharmacol 2012;7(3):214–28.
28. McCallum RW, Soykan I, Sridhar KR, et al. Delta-9-tetrahydrocannabinol delays the gastric emptying of solid food in humans: a double-blind, randomized study. Aliment Pharmacol Ther 1999;13:77–80.
29. Liu N, Abell T. Gastroparesis updates on pathogenesis and management. Gut Liver 2017;11:579–89.
30. Frantzides CT, Carlson MA, Zografakis JG, et al. Postoperative gastrointestinal complaints after laparoscopic Nissen fundoplication. JSLS 2006;10:39–42.
31. Nusrat S, Mahmood S, Kastens D, et al. Cholecystectomy for biliary dyskinesia in gastroparesis: mimic or misfortune? South Med J 2014;107(12):757–61.

32. Parkman HP, Yates K, Hasler WL, et al. Cholecystectomy and clinical presentations of gastroparesis. Dig Dis Sci 2013;58:1062–73.
33. Barboza JL, Okun MS, Moshiree B. The treatment of gastroparesis, constipation and small intestinal bacterial overgrowth syndrome in patients with Parkinson's disease. Expert Opin Pharmacother 2015;16:2449–64.
34. Goetze O, Nikodem AB, Wiezcorek J, et al. Predictors of gastric emptying in Parkinson's disease. Neurogastroenterol Motil 2006;18:369–75.
35. Doi H, Sakakibara R, Sato M, et al. Plasma levodopa peak delay and impaired gastric emptying in Parkinson's disease. J Neurol Sci 2012;319:86–8.
36. Raghav S, Kipp D, Watson J, et al. Gastroparesis with multiple sclerosis. Mult Scler 2006;12:243–4.
37. Chowdhury RS, Forsmark CE, Davis RH, et al. Prevalence of gastroparesis in patients with small duct chronic pancreatitis. Pancreas 2003;26:235–8.
38. Corral JE, Dye CW, Mascarenhas MR, et al. Is gastroparesis found more frequently in patients with cystic fibrosis? A systematic review. Scientifica (Cairo) 2016;2016:2918139.
39. Quigley EM. Other forms of gastroparesis: postsurgical, Parkinson, other neurologic diseases, connective tissue disorders. Gastroenterol Clin North Am 2015; 44:69–81.
40. Marie I, Gourcerol G, Leroi AM, et al. Delayed gastric emptying determined using the 13C-octanoic acid breath test in patients with systemic sclerosis. Arthritis Rheum 2012;64:2346–55.
41. Reinstein E, Pimentel M, Pariani M, et al. Visceroptosis of the bowel in the hypermobility type of Ehlers-Danlos syndrome: presentation of a rare manifestation and review of the literature. Eur J Med Genet 2012;55:548–51.
42. Hornbuckle K, Barnett JL. The diagnosis and work-up of the patient with gastroparesis. J Clin Gastroenterol 2000;30:117–24.
43. Waseem SH, Idrees MT, Croffie JM. Neuroenteric staining as a tool in the evaluation of pediatric motility disorders. Curr Gastroenterol Rep 2015;17:30.
44. Wadhwa V, Jobanputra Y, Thota PN, et al. Healthcare utilization and costs associated with cholangiocarcinoma. Gastroenterol Rep (Oxf) 2017;5:213–8.
45. Jones KL, Russo A, Berry MK, et al. A longitudinal study of gastric emptying and upper gastrointestinal symptoms in patients with diabetes mellitus. Am J Med 2002;113:449–55.
46. Horowitz M, Harding PE, Maddox AF, et al. Gastric and oesophageal emptying in patients with type 2 (non-insulin-dependent) diabetes mellitus. Diabetologia 1989;32:151–9.
47. Yu D, Ramsey FV, Norton WF, et al. The burdens, concerns, and quality of life of patients with gastroparesis. Dig Dis Sci 2017;62:879–93.
48. Wald A, Van Thiel DH, Hoechstetter L, et al. Gastrointestinal transit: the effect of the menstrual cycle. Gastroenterology 1981;80:1497–500.
49. Wang YR, Fisher RS, Parkman HP. Gastroparesis-related hospitalizations in the United States: trends, characteristics, and outcomes, 1995-2004. Am J Gastroenterol 2008;103:313–22.
50. Hammer J, Howell S, Bytzer P, et al. Symptom clustering in subjects with and without diabetes mellitus: a population-based study of 15,000 Australian adults. Am J Gastroenterol 2003;98:391–8.
51. Stanghellini V, Camilleri M, Malagelada JR. Chronic idiopathic intestinal pseudo-obstruction: clinical and intestinal manometric findings. Gut 1987;28:5–12.

52. Schatz RA, Zhang Q, Lodhia N, et al. Predisposing factors for positive D-Xylose breath test for evaluation of small intestinal bacterial overgrowth: a retrospective study of 932 patients. World J Gastroenterol 2015;21:4574–82.
53. Grover M, Farrugia G, Lurken MS, et al. Cellular changes in diabetic and idiopathic gastroparesis. Gastroenterology 2011;140:1575–85.e8.
54. Harberson J, Thomas RM, Harbison SP, et al. Gastric neuromuscular pathology in gastroparesis: analysis of full-thickness antral biopsies. Dig Dis Sci 2010;55: 359–70.
55. Bernard CE, Gibbons SJ, Mann IS, et al. Association of low numbers of CD206-positive cells with loss of ICC in the gastric body of patients with diabetic gastroparesis. Neurogastroenterol Motil 2014;26:1275–84.
56. Choi KM, Gibbons SJ, Nguyen TV, et al. Heme oxygenase-1 protects interstitial cells of Cajal from oxidative stress and reverses diabetic gastroparesis. Gastroenterology 2008;135:2055–64, 2064.e1-2.
57. Bharucha AE, Daley SL, Low PA, et al. Effects of hemin on heme oxygenase-1, gastric emptying, and symptoms in diabetic gastroparesis. Neurogastroenterol Motil 2016;28:1731–40.
58. Lin Z, Sarosiek I, Forster J, et al. Association of the status of interstitial cells of Cajal and electrogastrogram parameters, gastric emptying and symptoms in patients with gastroparesis. Neurogastroenterol Motil 2010;22:56–61, e10.
59. Gotfried J, Schey R. Understanding the differences between gastroparesis and gastroparesis-like syndrome: filling a GaPing hole? Dig Dis Sci 2017;62:2615–7.
60. Snape WJ, Lin MS, Agarwal N, et al. Evaluation of the pylorus with concurrent intraluminal pressure and EndoFLIP in patients with nausea and vomiting. Neurogastroenterol Motil 2016;28:758–64.
61. Friedenberg FK, Palit A, Parkman HP, et al. Botulinum toxin A for the treatment of delayed gastric emptying. Am J Gastroenterol 2008;103:416–23.
62. de la Loge C, Trudeau E, Marquis P, et al. Cross-cultural development and validation of a patient self-administered questionnaire to assess quality of life in upper gastrointestinal disorders: the PAGI-QOL. Qual Life Res 2004;13:1751–62.
63. Velanovich V. Difficulty in assessing quality of life outcomes in a fluctuating disease: a hypothesis based on gastroparesis. Gastroenterol Res Pract 2009; 2009:396190.
64. Pfeiffer RF. Gastrointestinal dysfunction in Parkinson's disease. Parkinsonism Relat Disord 2011;17(1):10–5.
65. Parkman HP, Yates K, Hasler WL, et al. Similarities and differences between diabetic and idiopathic gastroparesis. Clin Gastroenterol Hepatol 2011;9:1056–64 [quiz: e1133-1054].
66. Hasler WL, Wilson LA, Parkman HP, et al. Factors related to abdominal pain in gastroparesis: contrast to patients with predominant nausea and vomiting. Neurogastroenterol Motil 2013;25:427–38, e300-421.
67. Cherian D, Sachdeva P, Fisher RS, et al. Abdominal pain is a frequent symptom of gastroparesis. Clin Gastroenterol Hepatol 2010;8:676–81.
68. Bielefeldt K, Raza N, Zickmund SL. Different faces of gastroparesis. World J Gastroenterol 2009;15:6052–60.
69. Ananthakrishnan AN, Weber LR, Knox JF, et al. Permanent work disability in Crohn's disease. Am J Gastroenterol 2008;103:154–61.
70. Lu PL, Moore-Clingenpeel M, Yacob D, et al. The rising cost of hospital care for children with gastroparesis: 2004-2013. Neurogastroenterol Motil 2016;28:1698–704.
71. Kong MF, Horowitz M, Jones KL, et al. Natural history of diabetic gastroparesis. Diabetes Care 1999;22:503–7.

Diabetic Gastroparesis and Nondiabetic Gastroparesis

Shanshan Shen, MD, PhD[a], Jennifer Xu, MD[b], Vladimir Lamm, MD[b],
Cicily T. Vachaparambil, MD[b], Huimin Chen, MD, PhD[c], Qiang Cai, MD, PhD[b],*

KEYWORDS

- Gastroparesis • Etiology • Gastric peroral endoscopic pyloromyotomy (G-POEM)
- Peroral endoscopic pyloromyotomy (POP)

KEY POINTS

- Gastroparesis can be divided into diabetic gastroparesis and nondiabetic gastroparesis.
- Delayed gastric emptying is the main manifestation of motility disorders of both diabetic gastroparesis and nondiabetic gastroparesis.
- Symptoms of gastroparesis are nonspecific and the severity can vary.
- Gastric peroral endoscopic pyloromyotomy (G-POEM) brings more option for the treatment of diabetic and nondiabetic gastroparesis.

INTRODUCTION

Gastroparesis is defined as a syndrome of objectively delayed gastric emptying in the absence of mechanical obstruction. Characteristic symptoms of gastroparesis include early satiety, nausea, vomiting, bloating, and upper abdominal pain.[1] Gastroparesis has a significant impact on quality of life and increases the economic burden to family and society. In the United States, the number of emergency department visits and charges for a primary diagnosis of gastroparesis rose significantly from 2006 to 2013.[2] The number of hospitalizations increased from approximately 900 in 1994 to 16,440 in 2014.

Gastroparesis can be diabetic or nondiabetic. It is one of the well-known complications of longstanding diabetes that occurs in both type 1 diabetes mellitus and type 2 diabetes mellitus, and diabetes accounts for approximately one-third of

Disclosure Statement: The authors have no relevant commercial or financial conflicts of interest.
[a] Department of Gastroenterology, Nanjing Drum Tower Hospital, The Affiliated Hospital of Nanjing University Medical School, 321 Zhongshan Road, Nanjing 210008, China;
[b] Division of Digestive Diseases, Emory University, 1365 Clifton Road, Atlanta, GA 30322, USA;
[c] Division of Gastroenterology and Hepatology, Renji Hospital, School of Medicine, Shanghai Jiao Tong University, 160 Pujian Road, Shanghai 200127, China
* Corresponding author.
E-mail address: qcai@emory.edu

cases of gastroparesis. Nondiabetic causes include gastric surgery, drugs, neurologic disorders, connective tissue disease, and mesenteric ischemia. Approximately half of cases occur without a known etiology (idiopathic).[3] The complex etiologies and varied clinical features suggest a heterogenous pathogenesis. This article discusses the current research and features of both diabetic and nondiabetic gastroparesis.

ETIOLOGY OF DIABETIC AND NONDIABETIC GASTROPARESIS

The etiology of gastroparesis is diverse (**Box 1**). According to an epidemiologic study in Olmsted County, Minnesota, from 1996 to 2006, causes included 25.3% diabetes mellitus, 22.9% drugs, 10.8% connective tissue disease, 7.2% postsurgical gastroparesis (PSG), and 2.4% malignancy. Idiopathic gastroparesis was the cause in 49.4% of cases.[3] Delayed gastric emptying can be observed in 28% to 65% of unselected patients with diabetes. Women have slower gastric emptying than men.[4,5] On the basis of available epidemiologic data, compared with type 2 diabetics, patients with type 1 diabetes mellitus have a higher incidence of gastroparesis (5.2% in type 1 diabetes mellitus and 1% in type 2 diabetes mellitus) and earlier age of onset.[1] Type 2 diabetics, however, have more serious symptoms.[6] Gastroparesis in diabetic patients usually occurs 10 years after the onset of diabetes and in parallel with other forms of diabetic microvascular disease, including neuropathy, retinopathy, and so forth. Severe symptoms of diabetic gastroparesis cause poor glycemic control and poor nutritional status and increase the risk of hypoglycemia.

Several different etiologies contribute to nondiabetic gastroparesis. PSG with vagotomy or vagus nerve injury has become a recognized complication of operation at the upper abdomen.[1] The incidence of PSG after gastrectomy is approximately 0.4% to 5.0%. In the early postoperative period after pylorus-preserving pancreatoduodenectomy, PSG occurs in 20% to 50% of patients.[7] Another study reported that 67% of patients who underwent pancreatic cancer cryoablation and 5.1% after pancreatoduodenectomy were found with PSG.[8] Overall, the incidence of PSG depends on the surgical procedure and surgical site. Connective tissue disorders also may contribute to gastroparesis. For example, 50% to 75% of scleroderma patients with gastrointestinal symptoms have delayed gastric emptying with electrogastrogram (EGG) disturbances as high as 81.82%.[9,10] Idiopathic gastroparesis accounts for a large proportion and usually occurs in young women and patients who are overweight. Approximately one-fifth of idiopathic gastroparesis reported an initial infectious prodrome, suggesting virus may play a key role in the pathogenesis of gastroparesis.[11]

Box 1
The etiology of gastroparesis

Diabetic gastroparesis

Nondiabetic gastroparesis
  PSG (eg, gastrectomy)
  Nervous system disease (eg, parkinsonism)
  Connective tissue disease (eg, scleroderma)
  Idiopathic gastroparesis
  Paraneoplastic
  Mesenteric ischemia

MOTILITY DISORDERS OF DIABETIC AND NONDIABETIC GASTROPARESIS
Physiology of Normal Gastric Emptying

Gastric emptying refers to the process by which stomach contents are smoothly discharged into the duodenum. This process relies on the well-coordinated movement of stomach and duodenal smooth muscle. Smooth muscle, extrinsic and intrinsic neurons, glial cells, hormonal elements, and the interstitial cells of Cajal (ICCs) play an important role in this process.

Under normal circumstances, digestion grinds food into chime, which discharges into the duodenum, a process that lasts approximately 2 hours. This process consists of 4 steps: receiving, mixing, grinding, and emptying. The proximal stomach serves as the reservoir of food and the distal stomach as the grinder. When the food enters the stomach, the proximal stomach generates receptive relaxation and gastric pressure decreases, which are mediated by vagus nerve fibers. Then, slow and sustained contraction of the proximal stomach increases gastric cavity pressure and promotes gastric emptying. The process of gastric emptying is primarily regulated by the autonomic nervous system (especially the vagus nerve) and gastrointestinal hormones.

Gastric emptying scintigraphy at 15-minute intervals for 4 hours after food intake is considered the gold-standard for measuring gastric emptying in detail. Postprandial electrogastrogram (EGG) abnormalities may also predict delayed emptying of the stomach. Patients with delayed gastric emptying have a lower percentage of normal gastric slow waves and a significantly reduced increase of the dominant power in the postprandial EGG.[12]

The Relation Between Gastric Emptying and Hyperglycemia

Hyperglycemia has an important effect on gastric emptying. Although both delayed and rapid gastric emptying can be observed in diabetes mellitus, delayed gastric emptying occurs more frequently than rapid emptying.[13] Two-thirds of patients with poorly controlled type 2 diabetes mellitus have mostly asymptomatic yet abnormal gastric emptying.[14] Changes in blood glucose may slow gastric emptying in both diabetic and nondiabetic patients.[15,16] Acute hyperglycemia decreases fundic tone and contractility of the mid stomach and distal stomach and also alters small bowel contractile activity.[17] The stimulation of local pyloric contractions and inhibition of antral contractions contribute to the delayed gastric emptying induced by hyperglycemia.[18] The generation of gastric myoelectrical disturbances (in particular, tachygastria) was more prevalent during hyperglycemia.[19] On the contrary, insulin-induced hypoglycemia increases the gastric emptying rate in patients with type 1 diabetes mellitus.[20] This may reflect the self-regulation process of the body: when blood glucose falls, the gastric emptying increases to quickly absorb the nutrients and self-corrects for hypoglycemia.

Gastroparesis can make diabetes more difficult to manage. Gastric emptying is an important process in the regulation of blood glucose. Delayed emptying could worsen postprandial hypoglycemia in insulin-treated patients.[17] Furthermore, changes in gastric emptying may contribute to fluctuations in blood glucose.

Cellular Changes Contribute to Disorders of Gastric Emptying

On full-thickness biopsies, cellular abnormalities, including decreased ICCs, an abnormal immune infiltrate containing macrophages, and decreased nerve fibers are found in a majority of patients with diabetic and nondiabetic gastroparesis.[21] The intermyenteric plexus of muscularis propria from diabetic patients has fewer ganglia and ganglion cells than patients with idiopathic gastroparesis; however, the lymphocytic infiltrate and the loss of ICCs were not significantly different between diabetic and idiopathic gastroparesis.[22] These pathologic changes have considerable differences in the regional distribution.

Full-thickness pyloric and antral biopsies of 17 patients with gastroparesis showed that loss of ICCs in the pylorus is twice as common as in the antrum, and fibrosis in the pyloric smooth muscle is approximately 3 times more common than in the antrum.[23] These results implicate pyloric dysfunction in the pathologic process of gastroparesis.

ICCs are a special type of interstitial cells located between the gastrointestinal nerve endings and the smooth muscle. ICCs are pacemaker cells for slow waves to promote gastrointestinal motility. Kit immunolabeling has shown that ICC populations are impaired in both diabetic gastroparesis and nondiabetic gastroparesis patients. The absence of ICCs is associated with increased abnormalities of gastric slow waves, delayed gastric emptying, worse clinical symptoms, and poorer symptomatic response to gastric electrical stimulation (GES).[24–26] Recent studies illustrate possible mechanisms that can regulate ICCs networks in gastroparesis. Insulin and insulin-like growth factor 1 (IGF-1) receptors are detected in smooth muscle cells, which can promote the production of stem cell factor. Stem cell factor is essential for the development and maintenance of ICCs and its deficiency in diabetes is detrimental to ICCs.[27,28] An increased level of oxidative stress caused by low levels of heme oxygenase 1 (HO-1) is another possible etiology of ICC death. One study showed that inhibition of HO-1 activity in mice with normal gastric emptying causes a loss of Kit expression and development of diabetic gastroparesis.[29] The knockout of macrophage colony-stimulating factor (Csf1) in diabetic mice may reverse the reduction of ICCs and normalize gastric emptying, demonstrating that macrophages are necessary for the reduction of ICCs and the development of delayed gastric emptying.[30] The reduction of ICCs in nondiabetic gastroparesis has not yet been elucidated, and further research is needed to explore the mechanism of ICCs reduction in different types of gastroparesis.

Immune cells may play a role in development of gastroparesis. Full-thickness antral biopsies show an inflammatory infiltrate in approximately half of patients with diabetic gastroparesis.[31] In another histologic analysis, there is an overall 25% increase in CD45 (a marker of immune infiltrate) expression in diabetic gastroparesis and a 30% increase in CD45 in idiopathic gastroparesis compared with those of controls.[24]

M2 macrophages exert anti-inflammatory effects through induction of HO-1 to protect the ICCs network and thereby prevent the development of diabetic gastroparesis.[32] Both diabetic and idiopathic gastroparesis patients lose CD206$^+$ cells (M2 macrophages) in circular muscle and myenteric plexus, which also are associated with ICCs loss.[33] Another study showed a significant correlation between the number of CD206$^+$ cells and ICCs in diabetic gastroparesis but not in idiopathic gastroparesis.[34]

Nerve fiber loss is observed in both diabetic gastroparesis (17%) and idiopathic gastroparesis (14%) patients. Histologic and immunohistochemical studies of the resected specimen of idiopathic gastroparesis show hypoganglionosis and neuronal dysplasia.[35] Electron microscopy of enteric nerves from full-thickness stomach biopsies, showing a thickened basal lamina around smooth muscle cells and nerves is characteristic of diabetic gastroparesis whereas idiopathic gastroparesis has fibrosis, especially around nerves.[36] A decrease in number of nitric oxide synthase–positive neurons was also found in diabetic and idiopathic gastroparesis, with more severe reduction in idiopathic gastroparesis.[21] In animal tests, neuronal nitric oxide synthase–deficient mice show delayed gastric emptying of solids and liquids.[37]

Other Possible Pathogenesis of Gastroparesis

The sympathetic and parasympathetic nervous systems innervate the gastrointestinal movement by controlling motor, sensory, and secretory responses. Vagal nerve injury after surgery, such as gastrectomy, can cause PSG. In diabetic gastroparesis, autonomic neuropathy can affect sympathetic trunks and manifest as severe loss of myelinated fibers.[32] Diseases affecting the extrinsic neural control, such as parkinsonism, amyloidosis, and paraneoplastic disease, may contribute to gastroparesis. Some medications, including opiate analgesics, anticholinergic agents, and diabetes medications, may cause delayed gastric emptying.[1] The pathogenesis of these etiologies of gastroparesis, however, has not been clarified.

CLINICAL FEATURES OF DIABETIC AND NONDIABETIC GASTROPARESIS
Symptoms of Patients with Diabetic and Nondiabetic Gastroparesis

A tertiary referral study shows severity ranking of symptoms as follows: abdominal fullness, bloating, nausea, upper abdominal discomfort, upper abdominal pain, and vomiting[38]; however, these symptoms vary depending on etiology. In a study, including 157 patients (43 diabetic and 114 idiopathic), vomiting severity score and number of vomiting episodes were more severe in diabetic gastroparesis compared with idiopathic gastroparesis. Nausea is similar in all patients with gastroparesis, however, irrespective of cause. Both nausea and vomiting had a significant correlation with reduced quality of life.[39] One multicenter study showed that patients with diabetic gastroparesis had more severe retching and vomiting than those with idiopathic gastroparesis, whereas patients with idiopathic gastroparesis had more severe early satiety and postprandial fullness.[40] Another multicenter study of 393 patients showed abdominal pain was more prevalent with idiopathic gastroparesis and with lack of infectious prodrome compared with diabetic gastroparesis.[41] Early satiety and postprandial fullness are also common severe symptoms in both diabetic and idiopathic gastroparesis. Those symptoms are associated with other gastroparesis symptom severities, decrease in quality of life, and delayed gastric emptying.[42] Gastric hypersensitivity is increased in refractory diabetic gastroparesis, which could overstate symptoms, such as abdominal distension and fullness in patients with diabetic gastroparesis.[43]

The relationship between symptom and gastric emptying is uncertain. Surprisingly a meta-regression analysis did not find a significant relationship between symptom improvement and acceleration of gastric emptying with different drugs used for the treatment of gastroparesis.[44] Other studies, however, found that patients of idiopathic gastroparesis with severely delayed gastric emptying had worse vomiting and more severe loss of appetite and overall gastroparesis symptoms.[11] Some patients exhibit symptoms of gastroparesis but have normal or rapid emptying. Researchers believe these patients should also be classified on a spectrum of gastroparesis, which is called gastroparesis-like syndrome.[45] Pathophysiologic features of chronic unexplained nausea and vomiting, including loss of ICCs, are similar to those of gastroparesis, indicating that they could be spectra of the same disorder.[46]

Treatment of Diabetic and Nondiabetic Gastroparesis

Pharmacotherapy
Currently no drugs target underlying mechanisms of gastroparesis, with relief of symptoms the main purpose of medical treatment. Prokinetic medications are the most commonly used type of drug for the treatment of gastroparesis. Metoclopramide and domperidone are dopamine-2 receptor antagonists, which accelerate gastric

emptying and reduce symptoms of diabetic gastroparesis.[47,48] Antiemetics, such as prochlorperazine, ondansetron, diphenhydramine, and aprepitant, are all used as therapeutic drugs; however, there is no conclusive evidence for their effectiveness. For diabetic gastroparesis, the optimal glycemic control, which includes lifestyle modification and medication adherence, is the most important treatment option. Medications that can cause delayed gastric emptying, including opiates and anticholinergics, should be avoided in diabetic gastroparesis if possible. In the treatment of idiopathic gastroparesis and gastroparesis of other causes, effective drugs remain to be further studied.

Gastric electrical stimulation

GES involves delivering electric current via electrodes to gastric smooth muscle. GES with a high-frequency (12 cpm), low-energy (pulse width 330 microseconds) output was approved by the Food and Drug Administration in 2000 as a humanitarian device exemption for patients with refractory symptoms of diabetic or idiopathic gastroparesis. Evidence shows that diabetic gastroparesis has a better clinical response than idiopathic gastroparesis.[49] GES significantly decreases vomiting frequency and gastrointestinal symptoms and improves quality of life in diabetics with refractory gastroparesis; however, this is not the case in patients with idiopathic gastroparesis.[50] A meta-analysis, which includes 10 studies, suggests that diabetic gastroparesis patients seem most responsive to GES, whereas idiopathic gastroparesis patients and PSG patients are less responsive and need further research.[51] One possible explanation for the difference in response to GES is differences in the main symptoms experienced with gastroparesis. Patients with diabetic gastroparesis with mainly nausea/vomiting had a greater improvement than patients with idiopathic gastroparesis with mainly abdominal pain.[49] In patients with diabetic gastroparesis, GES also had a positive effect on metabolic control, with improvement in Hemoglobin A1c (HbA1c).[52] Based on a systematic review, the evidence in support of GES is limited and heterogeneous in quality.[53] The treatment of gastroparesis with GES remains controversial.

Gastric peroral endoscopic pyloromyotomy

Gastric peroral endoscopic pyloromyotomy (G-POEM), or peroral endoscopic pyloromyotomy (POP), is a novel treatment option for refractory gastroparesis based on the techniques and principles of esophageal per oral endoscopic myotomy, which was traditionally used for the management of achalasia. The procedure uses endoscopy to perform a pyloromyotomy. G-POEM, although technically more challenging than peroral endoscopic myotomy (POEM) because of its location, is a minimally invasive therapy. Multiple studies have shown the G-POEM is safe for patients with gastroparesis with symptoms refractory to medical therapy. Both diabetic gastroparesis and nondiabetic gastroparesis patients may benefit from G-POEM.[54] In 2013, the first human G-POEM in a 27-year-old woman with severe refractory diabetic gastroparesis symptoms was reported.[55] After the procedure, symptoms were significantly improved although gastric emptying remained delayed. Since then, there have been several studies suggesting that the G-POEM technique is both safe and effective and has an impact on both symptoms and gastric emptying. A small single-center noncontrolled study, which enrolled 16 patients, shows significant improvement in overall symptoms and gastric emptying after G-POEM, with no adverse events.[56] Recently, in a nonrandomized multicenter study, 30 patients (11 diabetic, 12 postsurgical, and 7 idiopathic) with gastroparesis receiving G-POEM were studied. Clinical response was remarkable in 86% of patients.[54] In univariate analysis of another study, diabetes and female gender were significantly associated with risk of failure.[57]

Although current evidence suggests efficacy, high-quality, large clinical trials are needed to establish the efficacy of G-POEM in patients with diabetic gastroparesis and nondiabetic gastroparesis.[58,59]

Prognostic Factors

The Gastroparesis Cardinal Symptom Index (GCSI), which was developed by Revicki and colleagues,[60] is a reliable and valid instrument for measuring symptom severity and to evaluate prognosis. Using GCSI, poor prognostic factors in both diabetic gastroparesis and idiopathic gastroparesis include increased body mass index or obesity, a history of smoking, use of pain modulators, moderate to severe abdominal pain, severe gastroesophageal reflex, and moderate to severe depression.[61] In idiopathic gastroparesis, female gender and being overweight may portend more severe symptoms.[11] Overall, in a follow-up period of approximately 25 years, diabetic gastroparesis is not associated with a poor prognosis or increased mortality.[62]

DISCUSSION

Gastroparesis is a functional disorder, which not only has an impact on quality of life but also increases economic burden to family and society. Gastroparesis can be categorized into diabetic and nondiabetic etiologies. Idiopathic gastroparesis accounts for a large proportion of nondiabetic gastroparesis. The incidence of gastroparesis depends significantly on etiology. Diabetes accounts for approximately one-third of cases, whereas morbidity of nondiabetic gastroparesis varies based on the specific causes.

Gastroparesis occurs more often in female patients. The symptom spectrum is similar between diabetic and nondiabetic gastroparesis, including nausea, vomiting, bloating, abdominal fullness, and abdominal pain. Whereas patients with diabetic gastroparesis have more severe vomiting and nausea, patients with idiopathic gastroparesis patients generally have earlier satiety and excessive abdominal fullness. The relationship between symptoms and gastric emptying is unsettled. The concept of a spectrum of gastroparesis (gastroparesis-like syndrome) adds to the mystery. Abnormalities of cytology and regulatory factors, including ICCs and IGF-1, have been found in both diabetic gastroparesis and nondiabetic gastroparesis. These irregularities provide not only a valuable basis for the diagnosis of gastroparesis but also new directions to guide research for treatment.

REFERENCES

1. Camilleri M, Parkman HP, Shafi MA, et al. Clinical guideline: management of gastroparesis. Am J Gastroenterol 2013;108(1):18–37 [quiz: 38].
2. Hirsch W, Nee J, Ballou S, et al. Emergency department burden of gastroparesis in the United States, 2006 to 2013. J Clin Gastroenterol 2017. https://doi.org/10.1097/MCG.0000000000000972.
3. Jung HK, Choung RS, Locke GR 3rd, et al. The incidence, prevalence, and outcomes of patients with gastroparesis in Olmsted County, Minnesota, from 1996 to 2006. Gastroenterology 2009;136(4):1225–33.
4. Samsom M, Vermeijden JR, Smout AJ, et al. Prevalence of delayed gastric emptying in diabetic patients and relationship to dyspeptic symptoms: a prospective study in unselected diabetic patients. Diabetes Care 2003;26(11):3116–22.
5. Jones KL, Russo A, Stevens JE, et al. Predictors of delayed gastric emptying in diabetes. Diabetes Care 2001;24(7):1264–9.

6. Horvath VJ, Izbeki F, Lengyel C, et al. Diabetic gastroparesis: functional/morphologic background, diagnosis, and treatment options. Curr Diab Rep 2014;14(9):527.

7. Dong K, Yu XJ, Li B, et al. Advances in mechanisms of postsurgical gastroparesis syndrome and its diagnosis and treatment. Chin J Dig Dis 2006;7(2):76–82.

8. Dong K, Li B, Guan QL, et al. Analysis of multiple factors of postsurgical gastroparesis syndrome after pancreaticoduodenectomy and cryotherapy for pancreatic cancer. World J Gastroenterol 2004;10(16):2434–8.

9. Quigley EM. Other forms of gastroparesis: postsurgical, Parkinson, other neurologic diseases, connective tissue disorders. Gastroenterol Clin North Am 2015; 44(1):69–81.

10. Marie I, Levesque H, Ducrotte P, et al. Gastric involvement in systemic sclerosis: a prospective study. Am J Gastroenterol 2001;96(1):77–83.

11. Parkman HP, Yates K, Hasler WL, et al. Clinical features of idiopathic gastroparesis vary with sex, body mass, symptom onset, delay in gastric emptying, and gastroparesis severity. Gastroenterology 2011;140(1):101–15.

12. Chen JD, Lin Z, Pan J, et al. Abnormal gastric myoelectrical activity and delayed gastric emptying in patients with symptoms suggestive of gastroparesis. Dig Dis Sci 1996;41(8):1538–45.

13. Kong MF, Horowitz M. Gastric emptying in diabetes mellitus: relationship to blood-glucose control. Clin Geriatr Med 1999;15(2):321–38.

14. Bharucha AE, Kudva Y, Basu A, et al. Relationship between glycemic control and gastric emptying in poorly controlled type 2 diabetes. Clin Gastroenterol Hepatol 2015;13(3):466–76.e461.

15. Schvarcz E, Palmer M, Aman J, et al. Physiological hyperglycemia slows gastric emptying in normal subjects and patients with insulin-dependent diabetes mellitus. Gastroenterology 1997;113(1):60–6.

16. Lysy J, Israeli E, Strauss-Liviatan N, et al. Relationships between hypoglycaemia and gastric emptying abnormalities in insulin-treated diabetic patients. Neurogastroenterol Motil 2006;18(6):433–40.

17. Kashyap P, Farrugia G. Diabetic gastroparesis: what we have learned and had to unlearn in the past 5 years. Gut 2010;59(12):1716–26.

18. Fraser R, Horowitz M, Dent J. Hyperglycaemia stimulates pyloric motility in normal subjects. Gut 1991;32(5):475–8.

19. Jebbink RJ, Samsom M, Bruijs PP, et al. Hyperglycemia induces abnormalities of gastric myoelectrical activity in patients with type I diabetes mellitus. Gastroenterology 1994;107(5):1390–7.

20. Schvarcz E, Palmer M, Aman J, et al. Hypoglycaemia increases the gastric emptying rate in patients with type 1 diabetes mellitus. Diabet Med 1993;10(7): 660–3.

21. Grover M, Farrugia G, Lurken MS, et al. Cellular changes in diabetic and idiopathic gastroparesis. Gastroenterology 2011;140(5):1575–85.e8.

22. Heckert J, Thomas RM, Parkman HP. Gastric neuromuscular histology in patients with refractory gastroparesis: relationships to etiology, gastric emptying, and response to gastric electric stimulation. Neurogastroenterol Motil 2017;29(8). https://doi.org/10.1111/nmo.13068.

23. Moraveji S, Bashashati M, Elhanafi S, et al. Depleted interstitial cells of Cajal and fibrosis in the pylorus: novel features of gastroparesis. Neurogastroenterol Motil 2016;28(7):1048–54.

24. Grover M, Bernard CE, Pasricha PJ, et al. Clinical-histological associations in gastroparesis: results from the Gastroparesis Clinical Research Consortium. Neurogastroenterol Motil 2012;24(6):531–9.e9.
25. Forster J, Damjanov I, Lin Z, et al. Absence of the interstitial cells of Cajal in patients with gastroparesis and correlation with clinical findings. J Gastrointest Surg 2005;9(1):102–8.
26. Lin Z, Sarosiek I, Forster J, et al. Association of the status of interstitial cells of Cajal and electrogastrogram parameters, gastric emptying and symptoms in patients with gastroparesis. Neurogastroenterol Motil 2010;22(1):56–61.e10.
27. Horvath VJ, Vittal H, Lorincz A, et al. Reduced stem cell factor links smooth myopathy and loss of interstitial cells of cajal in murine diabetic gastroparesis. Gastroenterology 2006;130(3):759–70.
28. Horvath VJ, Vittal H, Ordog T. Reduced insulin and IGF-I signaling, not hyperglycemia, underlies the diabetes-associated depletion of interstitial cells of Cajal in the murine stomach. Diabetes 2005;54(5):1528–33.
29. Choi KM, Gibbons SJ, Nguyen TV, et al. Heme oxygenase-1 protects interstitial cells of Cajal from oxidative stress and reverses diabetic gastroparesis. Gastroenterology 2008;135(6):2055–64, 2064.e1-2.
30. Cipriani G, Gibbons SJ, Verhulst PJ, et al. Diabetic Csf1(op/op) mice lacking macrophages are protected against the development of delayed gastric emptying. Cell Mol Gastroenterol Hepatol 2016;2(1):40–7.
31. Harberson J, Thomas RM, Harbison SP, et al. Gastric neuromuscular pathology in gastroparesis: analysis of full-thickness antral biopsies. Dig Dis Sci 2010;55(2):359–70.
32. Neshatian L, Gibbons SJ, Farrugia G. Macrophages in diabetic gastroparesis–the missing link? Neurogastroenterol Motil 2015;27(1):7–18.
33. Grover M, Bernard CE, Pasricha PJ, et al. Diabetic and idiopathic gastroparesis is associated with loss of CD206-positive macrophages in the gastric antrum. Neurogastroenterol Motil 2017;29(6). https://doi.org/10.1111/nmo.13018.
34. Bernard CE, Gibbons SJ, Mann IS, et al. Association of low numbers of CD206-positive cells with loss of ICC in the gastric body of patients with diabetic gastroparesis. Neurogastroenterol Motil 2014;26(9):1275–84.
35. Zarate N, Mearin F, Wang XY, et al. Severe idiopathic gastroparesis due to neuronal and interstitial cells of Cajal degeneration: pathological findings and management. Gut 2003;52(7):966–70.
36. Faussone-Pellegrini MS, Grover M, Pasricha PJ, et al. Ultrastructural differences between diabetic and idiopathic gastroparesis. J Cell Mol Med 2012;16(7):1573–81.
37. Mashimo H, Kjellin A, Goyal RK. Gastric stasis in neuronal nitric oxide synthase-deficient knockout mice. Gastroenterology 2000;119(3):766–73.
38. Cherian D, Sachdeva P, Fisher RS, et al. Abdominal pain is a frequent symptom of gastroparesis. Clin Gastroenterol Hepatol 2010;8(8):676–81.
39. Cherian D, Parkman HP. Nausea and vomiting in diabetic and idiopathic gastroparesis. Neurogastroenterol Motil 2012;24(3):217–22.e3.
40. Parkman HP, Yates K, Hasler WL, et al. Similarities and differences between diabetic and idiopathic gastroparesis. Clin Gastroenterol Hepatol 2011;9(12):1056–64 [quiz: e133–4].
41. Hasler WL, Wilson LA, Parkman HP, et al. Factors related to abdominal pain in gastroparesis: contrast to patients with predominant nausea and vomiting. Neurogastroenterol Motil 2013;25(5):427–38, e300-1.

42. Parkman HP, Hallinan EK, Hasler WL, et al. Early satiety and postprandial fullness in gastroparesis correlate with gastroparesis severity, gastric emptying, and water load testing. Neurogastroenterol Motil 2017;29(4). https://doi.org/10.1111/nmo.12981.

43. Phillips LK, Deane AM, Jones KL, et al. Gastric emptying and glycaemia in health and diabetes mellitus. Nat Rev Endocrinol 2015;11(2):112–28.

44. Janssen P, Harris MS, Jones M, et al. The relation between symptom improvement and gastric emptying in the treatment of diabetic and idiopathic gastroparesis. Am J Gastroenterol 2013;108(9):1382–91.

45. Liu N, Abell T. Gastroparesis updates on pathogenesis and management. Gut Liver 2017;11(5):579–89.

46. Angeli TR, Cheng LK, Du P, et al. Loss of interstitial cells of cajal and patterns of gastric dysrhythmia in patients with chronic unexplained nausea and vomiting. Gastroenterology 2015;149(1):56–66.e5.

47. Patterson D, Abell T, Rothstein R, et al. A double-blind multicenter comparison of domperidone and metoclopramide in the treatment of diabetic patients with symptoms of gastroparesis. Am J Gastroenterol 1999;94(5):1230–4.

48. McCallum RW, Ricci DA, Rakatansky H, et al. A multicenter placebo-controlled clinical trial of oral metoclopramide in diabetic gastroparesis. Diabetes Care 1983;6(5):463–7.

49. Maranki JL, Lytes V, Meilahn JE, et al. Predictive factors for clinical improvement with Enterra gastric electric stimulation treatment for refractory gastroparesis. Dig Dis Sci 2008;53(8):2072–8.

50. Abell T, McCallum R, Hocking M, et al. Gastric electrical stimulation for medically refractory gastroparesis. Gastroenterology 2003;125(2):421–8.

51. Chu H, Lin Z, Zhong L, et al. Treatment of high-frequency gastric electrical stimulation for gastroparesis. J Gastroenterol Hepatol 2012;27(6):1017–26.

52. van der Voort IR, Becker JC, Dietl KH, et al. Gastric electrical stimulation results in improved metabolic control in diabetic patients suffering from gastroparesis. Exp Clin Endocrinol Diabetes 2005;113(1):38–42.

53. Lal N, Livemore S, Dunne D, et al. Gastric electrical stimulation with the enterra system: a systematic review. Gastroenterol Res Pract 2015;2015:762972.

54. Khashab MA, Ngamruengphong S, Carr-Locke D, et al. Gastric per-oral endoscopic myotomy for refractory gastroparesis: results from the first multicenter study on endoscopic pyloromyotomy (with video). Gastrointest Endosc 2017; 85(1):123–8.

55. Khashab MA, Stein E, Clarke JO, et al. Gastric peroral endoscopic myotomy for refractory gastroparesis: first human endoscopic pyloromyotomy (with video). Gastrointest Endosc 2013;78(5):764–8.

56. Dacha S, Mekaroonkamol P, Li L, et al. Outcomes and quality-of-life assessment after gastric per-oral endoscopic pyloromyotomy (with video). Gastrointest Endosc 2017;86(2):282–9.

57. Gonzalez JM, Benezech A, Vitton V, et al. G-POEM with antro-pyloromyotomy for the treatment of refractory gastroparesis: mid-term follow-up and factors predicting outcome. Aliment Pharmacol Ther 2017;46(3):364–70.

58. Gonzalez JM, Lestelle V, Benezech A, et al. Gastric per-oral endoscopic myotomy with antropyloromyotomy in the treatment of refractory gastroparesis: clinical experience with follow-up and scintigraphic evaluation (with video). Gastrointest Endosc 2017;85(1):132–9.

59. Rodriguez JH, Haskins IN, Strong AT, et al. Per oral endoscopic pyloromyotomy for refractory gastroparesis: initial results from a single institution. Surg Endosc 2017;31(12):5381–8.
60. Revicki DA, Rentz AM, Dubois D, et al. Gastroparesis cardinal symptom index (GCSI): development and validation of a patient reported assessment of severity of gastroparesis symptoms. Qual Life Res 2004;13(4):833–44.
61. Pasricha PJ, Yates KP, Nguyen L, et al. Outcomes and factors associated with reduced symptoms in patients with gastroparesis. Gastroenterology 2015; 149(7):1762–74.e4.
62. Chang J, Rayner CK, Jones KL, et al. Prognosis of diabetic gastroparesis–a 25-year evaluation. Diabet Med 2013;30(5):e185–8.

Clinical Manifestation and Natural History of Gastroparesis

Priyadarshini Loganathan, MD[a], Mahesh Gajendran, MD, MPH[a],
Richard W. McCallum, FRACP (AUST)[b],*

KEYWORDS

- Gastroparesis • Natural history • Prognosis • Delayed gastric emptying • Nausea
- Vomiting • Quality of life • Mortality and morbidity

KEY POINTS

- Gastroparesis is a syndrome with delayed gastric emptying, resulting in symptoms without any evidence of obstruction in the upper gastrointestinal tract. The goal of evaluation is to exclude a mechanical obstruction and then establish the diagnosis of gastroparesis by an assessment of gastric motility.
- Nausea and vomiting are the cardinal symptoms of gastroparesis irrespective of etiology. The Gastroparesis Cardinal Symptom Index is a validated and reliable tool for assessing severity of symptoms associated with gastroparesis and to monitor treatment-induced changes in the symptoms of gastroparesis.
- The natural history to date suggests that over time gastric emptying in a majority of diabetic patients does not improve whereas in a majority of idiopathic gastroparesis patients it becomes faster or actually normalizes.

INTRODUCTION

Gastroparesis is a syndrome with delayed gastric emptying, resulting in symptoms without any evidence of obstruction in the upper gastrointestinal tract. The etiologies of gastroparesis are idiopathic, diabetes, postsurgical, autoimmune, and some neurologic conditions. Gastroparesis is a debilitating condition affecting more than 10 million patients, approximately 3% of US population. To give some perspective, celiac disease has 1% prevalence and hepatitis C has 2% to 3% prevalence. The

Disclosure of Funding: There is no source of funding involved in this study.
Conflict of interest statement: We declare that there is no conflict of interest.
[a] Department of Internal Medicine, Texas Tech University Health Sciences Center, Paul L. Foster School of Medicine, 4800 Alberta Avenue, El Paso, TX 79905, USA; [b] Division of Gastroenterology, Texas Tech University Health Sciences Center, Paul L Foster School of Medicine, 4800 Alberta Avenue, El Paso, TX 79905, USA
* Corresponding author.
E-mail address: Richard.mccallum@ttuhsc.edu

Gastrointest Endoscopy Clin N Am 29 (2019) 27–38
https://doi.org/10.1016/j.giec.2018.08.003
1052-5157/19/© 2018 Elsevier Inc. All rights reserved.

age-adjusted prevalence of gastroparesis per 100,000 persons is to be 9.6 (95% CI, 1.8–17.4) for men and 37.8 (95% CI, 23.3–52.4) for women.[1] Wang and colleagues[2] have showed that the hospitalization rates have increased in gastroparesis, implying increased prevalence as well as increased recognition and diagnosis of gastroparesis. This article elaborates on the clinical presentation of gastroparesis and its natural course. Much of the current understanding and knowledge about gastroparesis over the past 10 years is based on the contributions of the Gastroparesis Research Consortium, 7 academic centers funded by the National Institutes of Health to focus on the pathophysiology, diagnosis, treatment, and long-term follow-up of gastroparesis.

CLINICAL MANIFESTATION

Nausea and vomiting are the cardinal symptoms of gastroparesis irrespective of etiology (**Box 1**). The main clinical features of gastroparesis are nausea (>90% of patients), vomiting (68%–84% of patients), and feelings of fullness or early satiety after eating a small amount of food (50% of patients).[3–5] The pattern of vomiting poorly digested food that was eaten at least 1 hour to 12 hours earlier is often accompanied by acid reflux along with nausea, abdominal bloating, abdominal pain, changes in blood sugar levels, lack of appetite, weight loss, and malnutrition.[6] Bloating and abdominal pain are most likely due to sensory alteration,[7] whereas nausea, vomiting, early satiety, and postprandial fullness result from impaired smooth muscle and neural denervation, leading to delayed gastric emptying.[8] The clinical manifestations vary according to the etiology of the gastroparesis. Studies have shown that nausea and vomiting are more frequent in diabetic gastroparesis (DG) whereas abdominal pain is more observed in idiopathic gastroparesis (IG).[6,9]

The spectrum of disease ranges from mild to severe.[10] Waseem and colleagues[11] classified gastroparesis symptoms according to their severity: (1) mild gastroparesis: symptoms are easily controlled and patients are able to maintain their weight with minor dietary modification; (2) moderate gastroparesis: symptoms are frequent, although not present every day, and can be controlled with antiemetic and promotility agents along with diet and glucose control; while these gastroparesis patients are still able

---

Box 1
Common clinical presentation in gastroparesis

1. Nausea (93%)
2. Vomiting (68%–84%)
3. Early satiety (60%–86%)
4. Abdominal bloating (41%–76%)
5. Postprandial fullness
6. Lack of appetite
7. Abdominal pain (18%)
8. Heart burn/acid reflux
9. Weight loss
10. Malnutrition
11. Difficult glycemic control in diabetes

to work or sustain physical functions, there are intermittent emergency room visits and/or hospital admissions; and (3) severe gastroparesis: symptoms persist at a daily level despite maximum medical treatment, and there is accompanying malnutrition along with weight loss requiring frequent emergency room visits and multiple hospitalization. Their ability to function socially and professionally is affected and many patients are housebound and disabled by their symptoms. Homko and colleagues showed that even though the gastroparesis patients consumed and expended less calories compared with healthy controls, they were able to maintain neutral energy balance (intake calories = calories expended).[12]

Obesity has been identified as one of the possible contributors to gastroparesis, although the mechanism is unclear. Based on national data, greater than 35% of the US population has a body mass index of more than 35 kg/m^2 and some of these patients develop IG.[13] In 1 of the studies from the Gastroparesis Clinical Research Consortium (GpCRC), most of the IG patients were found to have either normal body weight (47%) or be overweight/obese (46%). Only 8% of the patients with IG were underweight. The cause of obesity in IG is unclear; however, 30% of the overweight patients were losing weight at the time of study enrollment.[10] Patients who were overweight had elevated inflammatory markers compared with normal weight patients, which led to the hypothesis that the ongoing inflammation could have been a contributory factor to the development of gastroparesis in these patients. Another side of this discussion of obesity and gastroparesis is the hypothesis that gastroenteritis illness can leads to IG in all patients, hence would occur in obese patients (>35% of US population) just as much as in normal weight patients.

In patients with type 2 diabetes mellitus, the obesity is often attributed to metabolic syndrome mostly present before DG symptoms begin. In a case-control study with diabetic neuropathy patients (N = 161), 83.2% of the cases were found to have at least 1 cardinal symptom of gastroparesis. In that study, obese patients reported significantly more early satiety (61.5% vs 35.2%; $P = .001$), fullness (63.7% vs 40.8%; $P = .004$), bloating (70.3% vs 49.3%; $P = .006$), and abdominal distention (71.4 vs 50.7%; $P = .007$) than nonobese subjects. This study suggests that obesity is an independent predictor of gastroparesis in patients with type 2 diabetes mellitus and neuropathy.[14]

It is important to evaluate for mood disorders in patients with gastroparesis. It has been found that approximately half of gastroparesis patients have moderate to severe depression as well as symptoms of anxiety.[15] Psychological illness is not the cause of gastric retention in these patients but psychological distress can worsen a patient's perception and grading of the symptom severity.[16] Psychiatric issues should be recognized and treated with appropriate pharmacologic therapy and psychotherapy, especially in refractory gastroparesis settings. It is debated, however, as to whether the depression is secondary to these patients having been searching for a diagnosis for some time in addition to having not received appropriate treatments. The incidence of physical and sexual abuse in IG patients has been reported to be greater than 30%. This sets the stage for higher abdominal pain prevalence in these patients and also contributes to the coexistence of irritable bowel syndrome and functional dyspepsia in gastroparesis patients.[5] Because women dominate in all of these entities, similar backgrounds are not a surprise.

Postsurgical gastroparesis (PSG) is a condition with chronic postoperative gastric atony in the absence of obstruction. PSG should be suspected in patients with persistent dyspeptic symptoms beginning soon after a surgical procedure, such as Billroth I and II antral resections, Roux-en-Y gastrojejunostomy, fundoplication, bariatric surgery involving pouches and gastrojejunostomy, esophagectomy with colonic interpositions or gastric pull-up, pylorus-preserving Whipple procedure, and lung transplantation.[17] Currently the most common surgical procedure resulting in gastroparesis is a Nissen fundoplication. In a prospective observational study of 615 patients who underwent laparoscopic Nissen fundoplication, a high incidence of temporary postoperative gastrointestinal symptoms suggestive of gastroparesis was documented. In the first 3 postoperative months, 88% of these patients had early satiety and 64% had bloating/flatulence. These symptoms are usually attributed to the gas-bloat syndrome—a well-known postfundoplication outcome because there is less belching due to impaired lower sphincter relaxation. By the end of 12 months, 90% of these patients were symptom-free.[18] The remaining group with chronic symptoms had gastroparesis attributed to damage to the vagus nerve by cautery, retraction, wrapping, or entrapping during the surgery and the most common vagus nerve that is generally affected is the left vagus nerve, which in turn becomes the anterior vagus nerve in the abdomen. Compared with DG or IG, patients with PSG have greater symptoms of early satiety, fullness, and bloating but less abdominal pain. The finding of bezoar on endoscopy is also more frequent in this subgroup.

DIAGNOSTIC CRITERIA

When gastroparesis is suspected, the goal of evaluation is to exclude a mechanical obstruction and then establish a diagnosis of gastroparesis by an assessment of gastric motility (**Fig. 1**). Thorough history and physical examination, including trying to elicit a succussion splash in the epigastric area, to rule out gastric outlet obstruction is important. Gastroparesis diabeticorum is an unique term first introduced by Kassander,[19] where patients have delayed gastric emptying without any symptoms of gastroparesis, and retained food was observed in the stomach during the upper gastrointestinal series. Esophagogastroduodenoscopy (EGD) can assess the pylorus stenosis as well as detect retained food, termed *bezoar*, in the stomach as an indicator for gastroparesis. In addition to an EGD, a small bowel follow-through barium study to exclude more distal problems, including superior mesenteric artery syndrome and malrotation of small bowel, is necessary.

The Gastroparesis Cardinal Symptom Index (GCSI) is a validated and reliable tool for assessing severity of symptoms associated with gastroparesis and to monitor treatment induced changes in the symptoms of gastroparesis (**Table 1**).[20] It has 3 subscales: postprandial fullness/early satiety (4 items), nausea/vomiting (3 items), and bloating (2 items). Reviki and colleagues[21] showed that the GCSI scores correlated well with the gastroparesis symptom severity, as rated by clinicians ($P<.0001$) and patients ($P = .0004$). Criteria generally used for entry into clinical trials usually require a GCSI score greater than 2.5 consistent with mild to moderate severity.

The most widely available technique to confirm the presence of delayed gastric emptying time is gastric emptying scintigraphy. Solid-phase gastric emptying scintigraphy is used to document the gastroparesis whereas liquid-phase gastric emptying scintigraphy is not generally used because noncaloric liquid emptying is mostly preserved even in refractory gastroparesis.[22] Delayed gastric emptying is defined as greater than 90% of gastric retention at 1 hour, greater than 60% at 2 hours, greater than 30% at 3 hours, and greater than 10% at 4 hours after meal ingestion.

DIFFERENTIAL DIAGNOSIS

The differential diagnosis of gastroparesis includes other causes of chronic nausea and vomiting, including different conditions that could potentially be misdiagnosed

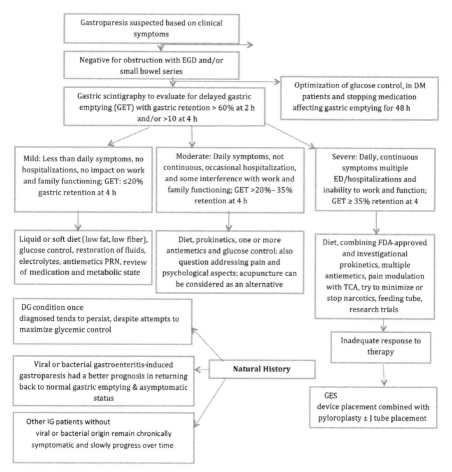

Fig. 1. Flow chart of gastroparesis is schematized. DG, diabetic gastroparesis; DM, diabetes mellitus; ED, emergency department; EGD, esophagogastroduodenoscopy; FDA, Food and Drug Administration; GES, gastric electrical stimulation; GET, gastric emptying time; IG, idiopathic gastroparesis; J tube, jejunostomy tube; PRN, as needed; TCA, tricyclic antidepressants.

Table 1	
Gastroparesis cardinal symptom index	
Symptom Subscale	**Symptom**
Nausea/vomiting	• Nausea • Retching • Vomiting
Postprandial fullness/early satiety	• Stomach fullness • Not able to finish normal-sized meal • Feeling excessively fullness after meals • Loss of appetite
Bloating/distention	• Bloating • Belly visibly larger

Graded from 0 to 5 (0 = none; 1 = very mild; 2 = mild; 3 = moderate; 4 = severe; and 5 = very severe) with a 2-week recall period.

From Revicki DA, Rentz AM, Dubois D, et al. Gastroparesis Cardinal Symptom Index [GCSI]: development and validation of a patient reported assessment of severity of gastroparesis symptoms. Qual Life Res 2004;13[4]:843; with permission.

or misinterpreted as gastroparesis and can make its diagnosis challenging. Some of the most commonly considered differential diagnoses are

1. Functional dyspepsia: functional dyspepsia symptoms often overlap with IG. It is further classified into (a) postprandial distress syndrome (PDS) featuring meal-induced fullness and satiety and (b) epigastric pain syndrome featuring epigastric pain and burning sensation, including a nocturnal timing on the fasted stomach.[23] The cardinal symptoms of nausea and vomiting in gastroparesis are less common in functional dyspepsia whereas gastric emptying study is generally normal; 20% to 40% of functional dyspepsia patients with PDS subtype can have delayed gastric emptying blurring its differentiation from gastroparesis. The abdominal pain in PDS subtype of functional dyspepsia is less than in the IG.[24]

2. Gastroparesis like syndrome: these patients with gastroparesis like syndrome have nausea and vomiting symptoms indistinguishable from gastroparesis, but they have normal gastric emptying study.[25] It is hypothesized that over time some of these patients, in particular diabetics, may eventually evolve and meet criteria for being diagnosed with gastroparesis.

3. Cyclic vomiting syndrome: vomiting episodes accompanied by severe epigastric pain can last for hours to days and are separated by symptom-free periods of variable lengths (months). It is usually associated with severe stress states, migraines, and diabetes. The key here is that the gastric emptying time is normal or rapid in the symptom-free period.

4. Cannabinoid hyperemesis syndrome: it is characterized by chronic cannabis use, cyclic episodes of nausea and vomiting, and frequent hot bathing. It is really a subset of the cyclic vomiting syndrome umbrella. Both conditions share the cycled attacks of vomiting and severe abdominal pain.

5. Rumination vomiting: a fountain-like regurgitation of undigested food occurs within 5 minutes to 25 minutes of food intake and is preceded by burping and belching. The onset of this syndrome is chronologically associated with severe stress and life-altering events.

6. Dumping syndrome: this occurs in approximately 20% of patients after vagotomy with pyloroplasty or distal gastrectomy, resulting in rapid emptying of hyperosmolar chyme into the small bowel. It is also seen in earlier stages of diabetes as well as idiopathic dumping syndrome group, where it is attributed to postviral damage to the duodenal mucosa or the vagus nerve. In early dumping, approximately 15 minutes to 30 minutes after a meal, patients experience abdominal discomfort, nausea, vomiting, and the vasomotor symptoms, whereas later symptoms are diarrhea, weakness, and fainting feelings from hypoglycemia. Gastric emptying study is rapid in the dumping syndrome.

7. Connective tissue disorders: Some patients who have been diagnosed with IG could have an underlying connective tissue disorder, most commonly systemic sclerosis. Hence, the finding of Raynaud syndrome should be sought along with Sjögren syndrome, gastric reflux, and dysphagia. Often entities that can mimic IG are infiltrative enteritis, amyloidosis, eosinophilic gastroenteritis, and autoimmune conditions, such as myasthenia gravis; demyelinating disease, such as multiple sclerosis; and paraneoplastic syndrome.[26,27]

8. Dysautonomia: the joint hypermobility syndrome, Ehlers-Danlos type 3, can be accompanied by postural orthostatic tachycardia syndrome. Approximately 30% of these patients have dysautonomia, which leads to either rapid or slow gastric emptying.[28]

9. Celiac axis compression syndrome/median arcuate ligament syndrome: it is defined as chronic, recurrent abdominal pain related to compression of the celiac

artery, specifically the celiac ganglion by the median arcuate ligament. This pain is out of proportion to any objective data or findings. The triad of postprandial abdominal pain, weight loss, and nausea and vomiting is characteristic of celiac axis compression syndrome.[29] An abdominal bruit occasionally may be auscultated.

NATURAL COURSE

Understanding the natural history of gastroparesis is still evolving. DG condition once diagnosed tends to persist, despite attempts to maximize glycemic control. Studies have shown that gastric emptying and symptoms are stable during greater than or equal to 12 years' follow-up, despite improved glycemic control.[30,31] Generally gastroparesis develops after having more than 5 years of diabetes, generally accompanied by microvascular complications from diabetes, such as retinopathy, nephropathy, or autonomic or peripheral neuropathy. Approximately 10% to 12% of these patients have type 1 diabetes mellitus. Conversely, Jones and colleagues[32] did not find any changes in gastric emptying or upper gastrointestinal symptoms over a decade of follow-up in diabetic patients. Bytzer and colleagues[33] studied 8657 eligible patients with diabetes and found increased prevalence of upper gastrointestinal symptoms with poor glycemic control, independent of duration or type of diabetes. Hyett and colleagues[34] reported increased morbidity in patients with DG with higher incidence of cardiovascular disease (19.2% vs 6.4%; $P<.05$), hypertension (63% vs 43%, $P = .005$), and retinopathy (33% vs 11.7%, $P<.001$) compared with diabetic patients with no gastroparesis symptoms. Also, diabetic patients with gastroparesis had more emergency room visits and frequent hospital admissions compared with diabetic patients with no symptoms of gastroparesis.[2,34]

In a study from the National Institutes of Health gastroparesis consortium GpCRC, 142 gastroparesis patients (36 DG and 106 IG) were reassessed at 48 weeks after the time of enrollment to determine the progression of the disease.[35] Overall, 15% of the patients had worsening of the gastric emptying defined as 12% or greater retention of isotope labeled meal at 4 hours compared with the baseline study; 42% had no change and 43% had improvement in gastric emptying. A greater proportion of patients with DG had worsening of gastric emptying time compared with IG (25% vs 12%). Predictors of improved gastric emptying include baseline narcotic use, initial increased gastric retention, less depression, more severe gastroesophageal reflux disease, and elevated C-reactive protein.[35] McCallum and colleagues reported viral gastroparesis as a subgroup of IG was characterized by acute-onset, initial severe illness followed by slow resolution toward a satisfactory quality of life (QOL).[36] Viral or bacterial gastroenteritis-induced gastroparesis had a better prognosis in returning to being asymptomatic status and their gastric emptying normalizing compared with DG. The group of IG without an obvious viral or bacterial origin seems more likely to remain stable or slowly progress and be symptomatic for a longer period of time.

A study conducted on 165 patients with gastroparesis found that gastric emptying in patients who were refractory to medical management were much slower than gastroparesis patients whose symptoms responded to medical management.[37] At least 25% fail the medical management and require gastric electric stimulation (GES), which improved gastroparesis symptoms and health care utilization in these patient groups.[38]

In PSG patients, gastroparesis symptoms may improve over time from surgery due to adaptation of enteral nervous system to the loss of vagal input or from regeneration of the remaining vagal nerve fibers in the setting that gastric emptying was actually normal before the surgery. If the symptoms persist over a year, the medical management would be more challenging and many of these patients refractory to available medical or surgical management. These patients may have chronic abdominal pain from the surgeries requiring narcotics. It is crucial to have a multidisciplinary care team, including nutritionist, psychologist, pain specialist, gastroenterologist, and primary physician, to manage these patients effectively.

Because several other conditions may mimic the diagnosis of gastroparesis, the impact of wrong diagnosis has a significant role in the prognosis and the natural history of the gastroparesis. Use of narcotics for pain control delays the gastric emptying time, which could lead to an incorrect diagnosis of gastroparesis as well as cause constipation and bloating. The coexisting use of marijuana also can worsen gastroparesis symptoms by delaying the gastric emptying time and making the treatment more difficult. If all medical measures fail, options for maintaining nutrition include placement of gastrostomy tube for gastric decompression and jejunostomy for enteral feeding.[39] A study by Soykan and colleagues[5] found that in 146 gastroparesis patients seen at a tertiary medical center, 21% of them required nutritional support (enteral or parenteral feeding) and 26% were considered nonresponders to prokinetic agents and eventually underwent surgical intervention (total gastrectomy or GES).

Patients with gastroparesis are at increased risk of dehydration and electrolyte, nutritional, and micronutrient abnormalities due to recurrent emesis and poor oral intake during the flare up. Due to chronic early satiety, patients develop aversion to food intake that eventually either results in weight loss or anorexia. In a prospective study of 156 gastroparesis patients in the GpCRC registry with 48 weeks' follow-up, 6.5% of the patients were started on total parental nutrition, 5% had placement of jejunostomy tube for enteral feeding, and 30.5% had placement of GES device.[40]

A retrospective study of approximately 10 years in patients with severe gastroparesis (N = 221) treated with GES showed that the total symptom score, hospitalization days, and the use of medications were significantly reduced among these patients.[41] In addition, 80% of patients who had required a feeding jejunostomy initially were able to have it removed after GES. Patients with diabetic gastroparesis DG and PSG experienced more benefit from GES than those with IG. The investigators concluded that the GES therapy significantly improved subjective and objective parameters in patients with severe gastroparesis, with sustained efficacy, safety, and tolerance profiles up to 10 years.[41] Despite the improvement in the symptoms with GES therapy, the acceleration of gastric emptying was unpredictable. These data and results lead to the decision to pursue the GES combined with pyloroplasty as the most logical approach to achieve significant acceleration of gastric emptying.

Laparoscopic pyloroplasty in selected gastroparesis patients improved the gastric emptying times with low morbidity.[42] Sarosiek and colleagues[43] compared gastroparesis patients who received GES therapy alone and those with both GES and surgical pyloroplasty with a 7-month follow-up. The total symptom score improved significantly in both groups compared with their baseline scores ($P<.001$). The gastric emptying improved, however, by 64% at 4 hours ($P < .001$) in patients with both GES and pyloroplasty compared with 7% in the GES-only group. The postvagotomy gastroparesis patients had the most impressive acceleration of gastric emptying and 60% of them had normal gastric emptying times.[43]

EFFECT ON QUALITY OF LIFE

Fatigue is an important and common symptom in gastroparesis, which results in lower QOL. In a study by Cherian and colleagues,[44] 93% of the gastroparesis patients (N = 156) reported fatigue measured by the fatigue assessment instrument. In that study, moderate correlations were seen between fatigue and upper abdominal discomfort (r = 0.446), upper abdominal pain (r = 0.422), loss of appetite (r = 0.329), bloating (r = 0.297), and abdominal distention (r = 0.265) in gastroparesis. Fatigue severity correlated with a decreased QOL (r = −0.694, P < .001), increased depression (r = 0.339, P = .009), lower anxiety (r = −0.441, P < .001), and lower hemoglobin levels (r = −0.258, P = .005). This possibly is explained by their decreased nutritional intake, specifically iron and vitamin B_{12}. There was no correlation between fatigue and glycosylated hemoglobin, erythrocyte sedimentation rate, C-reactive protein, thyroid-stimulating hormone, or gastric emptying.[44]

Patients with severe gastroparesis are associated with higher depression and anxiety scores. The psychological dysfunction did not vary, however, by etiology or degree of gastric retention. Also it is still unclear whether these psychological abnormalities are a cause or a consequence of severe gastrointestinal symptoms. Nevertheless, it is of paramount importance to factor in both physical and psychological features when developing individualized treatment plans for gastroparesis.[16] Studies have also shown improvement in QOL with psychological intervention in gastroparesis.[45]

Nausea is the most important symptom associated, with worse QOL measured by Patient Assessment of Gastrointestinal Disorders-Symptom Severity Index (PAGI-SYM) and Patient Assessment of Upper Gastrointestinal Disorders-Quality of Life (PAGI-QOL). DG and IG had similar nausea and vomiting scores but retching is more severe (2.6 ± 0.3 vs 1.4 ± 0.3; P = .02) with more episodes of vomiting per week in DG (4.4 ± 1.4 vs 3.5 ± 1.3; P = .037) compared with IG.[46]

Gastroparesis symptoms in diabetics were associated with significantly reduced QOL irrespective of their age, gender, smoking, alcohol use, and type of diabetes.[47] A questionnaire-based survey of 1423 gastroparesis patients revealed significantly decreased QOL as assessed by the 36-Item Short Form Health Survey, in particular the physical health component (social function and general health scores). The mental and emotional health scores were relatively good, given that these patients have a high incidence of anxiety and depression.[16,48] Physical health QOL score was negatively correlated with symptoms, including nausea (r = −0.37), upper abdominal pain (r = −0.37), and early satiety (r = −0.37). Thus, focusing on adequate management of these symptoms could effectively improve the overall QOL. Gastroparesis not only affects the QOL but also causes significant financial burden on the health care system.

MORTALITY RATES

The mortality in gastroparesis patients can be explained by the following factors: (1) gastroparesis-related complications, (2) complications from treatment of gastroparesis, and (3) underlying causes of gastroparesis. The median time of death in DG gastroparesis patients from the time of diagnosis of gastroparesis was 6 years (range 1–12). The data from Rochester Epidemiology Project with 5-year follow-up showed that the overall survival of gastroparesis patients was significantly lower than in the Minnesota white population, after adjusting for age and gender (67% vs 81%, P<.01).[1] The mortality in patients with DG is mainly due to the complications of other end organ damage. Also, Cutts and colleagues[38] showed higher mortality in patients who had severe symptomatic gastroparesis who were referred for gastric stimulator but did not undergo GES placement. Conversely, in a prospective cohort study in patients with long-standing diabetes, a majority of patients were alive after a period of 9 years to 14 years, and the risk of death was not increased with prolonged solid or liquid gastric emptying.[49] These findings were further confirmed by another prospective cohort study, in which most of the diabetic patients with delayed gastric emptying were alive after 25 years of follow-up.[50] Both of these later studies were conducted in an endocrinology unit by an endocrinologist and not in a gastroenterology referral setting.

SUMMARY

Although it has been more 60 years since gastroparesis has been described, there is limited knowledge available about its natural history. Community research on gastroparesis natural history has not been conducted, and tertiary center analysis may not be fully representative of the findings of the gastroparesis in general population. The natural course of gastroparesis may differ according to its etiology. It could start with abrupt initiation of its symptoms if due to an infectious etiology and in contrast to slowly progressive and prolonged symptoms in DG. The poor glycemic control, infection, noncompliance, or intolerance of medical treatment results in higher hospitalization rates. This natural history is viewed in the setting of limited treatment options. Metoclopramide is the only Food and Drug Administration (FDA)-approved drug since 1983 and there is a major reliance on antiemetics for symptomatic treatment in gastroparesis. Recently, there have been important advancements in knowledge about the underlying pathogenesis of gastroparesis, which have led to targeted therapies to improve the gastric motility, hence thereby improving the symptoms and quality of life in patients with gastroparesis.

REFERENCES

1. Jung HK, Choung RS, Locke GR 3rd, et al. The incidence, prevalence, and outcomes of patients with gastroparesis in Olmsted County, Minnesota, from 1996 to 2006. Gastroenterology 2009;136(4):1225–33.
2. Wang YR, Fisher RS, Parkman HP. Gastroparesis-related hospitalizations in the United States: trends, characteristics, and outcomes, 1995-2004. Am J Gastroenterol 2008;103(2):313–22.
3. Camilleri M, Parkman HP, Shafi MA, et al. Clinical guideline: management of gastroparesis. Am J Gastroenterol 2013;108(1):18–37 [quiz: 38].
4. Parkman HP, Hasler WL, Fisher RS, et al. American Gastroenterological Association technical review on the diagnosis and treatment of gastroparesis. Gastroenterology 2004;127(5):1592–622.
5. Soykan I, Sivri B, Sarosiek I, et al. Demography, clinical characteristics, psychological and abuse profiles, treatment, and long-term follow-up of patients with gastroparesis. Dig Dis Sci 1998;43(11):2398–404.
6. Cherian D, Sachdeva P, Fisher RS, et al. Abdominal pain is a frequent symptom of gastroparesis. Clin Gastroenterol Hepatol 2010;8(8):676–81.
7. Hasler WL, Wilson LA, Parkman HP, et al. Factors related to abdominal pain in gastroparesis: contrast to patients with predominant nausea and vomiting. Neurogastroenterol Motil 2013;25(5):427–38, e300-421.
8. Hasler WL, Wilson LA, Parkman HP, et al. Bloating in gastroparesis: severity, impact, and associated factors. Am J Gastroenterol 2011;106(8):1492–502.
9. Cherian D, Parkman HP. Nausea and vomiting in diabetic and idiopathic gastroparesis. Neurogastroenterol Motil 2012;24(3):217–22, e103.
10. Parkman HP, Yates K, Hasler WL, et al. Clinical features of idiopathic gastroparesis vary with sex, body mass, symptom onset, delay in gastric emptying, and gastroparesis severity. Gastroenterology 2011;140(1):101–15.
11. Waseem S, Moshiree B, Draganov PV. Gastroparesis: current diagnostic challenges and management considerations. World J Gastroenterol 2009;15(1):25–37.

12. Homko CJ, Zamora LC, Boden G, et al. Bodyweight in patients with idiopathic gastroparesis: roles of symptoms, caloric intake, physical activity, and body metabolism. Neurogastroenterol Motil 2014;26(2):283–9.
13. Flegal KM, Kruszon-Moran D, Carroll MD, et al. Trends in obesity among adults in the United States, 2005 to 2014. JAMA 2016;315(21):2284–91.
14. Boaz M, Kislov J, Dickman R, et al. Obesity and symptoms suggestive of gastroparesis in patients with type 2 diabetes and neuropathy. J Diabetes Complications 2011;25(5):325–8.
15. Talley SJ, Bytzer P, Hammer J, et al. Psychological distress is linked to gastrointestinal symptoms in diabetes mellitus. Am J Gastroenterol 2001;96(4):1033–8.
16. Hasler WL, Parkman HP, Wilson LA, et al. Psychological dysfunction is associated with symptom severity but not disease etiology or degree of gastric retention in patients with gastroparesis. Am J Gastroenterol 2010;105(11):2357–67.
17. Eagon JC, Miedema BW, Kelly KA. Postgastrectomy syndromes. Surg Clin North Am 1992;72(2):445–65.
18. Shafi MA, Pasricha PJ. Post-surgical and obstructive gastroparesis. Curr Gastroenterol Rep 2007;9(4):280–5.
19. Kassander P. Asymptomatic gastric retention in diabetics (gastroparesis diabeticorum). Ann Intern Med 1958;48(4):797–812.
20. Revicki DA, Rentz AM, Dubois D, et al. Development and validation of a patient-assessed gastroparesis symptom severity measure: the Gastroparesis Cardinal Symptom Index. Aliment Pharmacol Ther 2003;18(1):141–50.
21. Revicki DA, Rentz AM, Dubois D, et al. Gastroparesis Cardinal Symptom Index (GCSI): development and validation of a patient reported assessment of severity of gastroparesis symptoms. Qual Life Res 2004;13(4):833–44.
22. Chaudhuri TK, Fink S. Gastric emptying in human disease states. Am J Gastroenterol 1991;86(5):533–8.
23. Parkman HP, Camilleri M, Farrugia G, et al. Gastroparesis and functional dyspepsia: excerpts from the AGA/ANMS meeting. Neurogastroenterol Motil 2010;22(2):113–33.
24. Tack J, Talley NJ, Camilleri M, et al. Functional gastroduodenal disorders. Gastroenterology 2006;130(5):1466–79.
25. Pasricha PJ, Colvin R, Yates K, et al. Characteristics of patients with chronic unexplained nausea and vomiting and normal gastric emptying. Clin Gastroenterol Hepatol 2011;9(7):567–76.e1-4.
26. Sridhar KR, Lange RC, Magyar L, et al. Prevalence of impaired gastric emptying of solids in systemic sclerosis: diagnostic and therapeutic implications. J Lab Clin Med 1998;132(6):541–6.
27. Park K, Park S, Jackson MW. The inhibitory effects of antimuscarinic autoantibodies in the sera of primary Sjogren syndrome patients on the gastrointestinal motility. Mol Immunol 2013;56(4):583–7.
28. Fikree A, Aktar R, Grahame R, et al. Functional gastrointestinal disorders are associated with the joint hypermobility syndrome in secondary care: a case-control study. Neurogastroenterol Motil 2015;27(4):569–79.
29. Balaban DH, Chen J, Lin Z, et al. Median arcuate ligament syndrome: a possible cause of idiopathic gastroparesis. Am J Gastroenterol 1997;92(3):519–23.
30. Camilleri M, Bharucha AE, Farrugia G. Epidemiology, mechanisms, and management of diabetic gastroparesis. Clin Gastroenterol Hepatol 2011;9(1):5–12 [quiz: e17].
31. Rayner CK, Horowitz M. New management approaches for gastroparesis. Nat Clin Pract Gastroenterol Hepatol 2005;2(10):454–62 [quiz: 493].

32. Jones KL, Russo A, Berry MK, et al. A longitudinal study of gastric emptying and upper gastrointestinal symptoms in patients with diabetes mellitus. Am J Med 2002;113(6):449–55.
33. Bytzer P, Talley NJ, Leemon M, et al. Prevalence of gastrointestinal symptoms associated with diabetes mellitus: a population-based survey of 15,000 adults. Arch Intern Med 2001;161(16):1989–96.
34. Hyett B, Martinez FJ, Gill BM, et al. Delayed radionucleotide gastric emptying studies predict morbidity in diabetics with symptoms of gastroparesis. Gastroenterology 2009;137(2):445–52.
35. Parkman HP, McCallum R, Yates K, et al. Gatsric emptying changes over time in gastroparesis: Comparision of initial and 48 week follow up gastric emptying tests in teh gastroparesis registry of the gastroparesis consortium. Abstract In DDW. 2018.
36. Bityutskiy LP, Soykan I, McCallum RW. Viral gastroparesis: a subgroup of idiopathic gastroparesis–clinical characteristics and long-term outcomes. Am J Gastroenterol 1997;92(9):1501–4.
37. Hejazi RA, Sarosiek I, Roeser K, et al. Does grading the severity of gastroparesis based on scintigraphic gastric emptying predict the treatment outcome of patients with gastroparesis? Dig Dis Sci 2011;56(4):1147–53.
38. Cutts TF, Luo J, Starkebaum W, et al. Is gastric electrical stimulation superior to standard pharmacologic therapy in improving GI symptoms, healthcare resources, and long-term health care benefits? Neurogastroenterol Motil 2005;17(1):35–43.
39. McCallum R, Lin Z, Wetzel P, et al. Clinical response to gastric electrical stimulation in patients with postsurgical gastroparesis. Clin Gastroenterol Hepatol 2005; 3(1):49–54.
40. Pasricha PJ, Nguyen LAB, Snape WJ, et al. 1069 changes in quality of life and symptoms in a large cohort of patients with gastroparesis followed prospectively for 48 weeks. Gastroenterology 2010;138(5):S-155.
41. McCallum RW, Lin Z, Forster J, et al. Gastric electrical stimulation improves outcomes of patients with gastroparesis for up to 10 years. Clin Gastroenterol Hepatol 2011;9(4):314–9, e311.
42. Toro JP, Lytle NW, Patel AD, et al. Efficacy of laparoscopic pyloroplasty for the treatment of gastroparesis. J Am Coll Surg 2014;218(4):652–60.
43. Sarosiek I, Forster J, Lin Z, et al. The addition of pyloroplasty as a new surgical approach to enhance effectiveness of gastric electrical stimulation therapy in patients with gastroparesis. Neurogastroenterol Motil 2013;25(2):134.
44. Cherian D, Paladugu S, Pathikonda M, et al. Fatigue: a prevalent symptom in gastroparesis. Dig Dis Sci 2012;57(8):2088–95.
45. Woodhouse S, Hebbard G, Knowles SR. Psychological controversies in gastroparesis: a systematic review. World J Gastroenterol 2017;23(7):1298–309.
46. Jaffe JK, Paladugu S, Gaughan JP, et al. Characteristics of nausea and its effects on quality of life in diabetic and idiopathic gastroparesis. J Clin Gastroenterol 2011;45(4):317–21.
47. Talley NJ, Young L, Bytzer P, et al. Impact of chronic gastrointestinal symptoms in diabetes mellitus on health-related quality of life. Am J Gastroenterol 2001;96(1): 71–6.
48. Yu D, Ramsey FV, Norton WF, et al. The burdens, concerns, and quality of life of patients with gastroparesis. Dig Dis Sci 2017;62(4):879–93.
49. Kong MF, Horowitz M, Jones KL, et al. Natural history of diabetic gastroparesis Diabetes care 1999;22(3):503–7.
50. Chang J, Rayner CK, Jones KL, et al. Prognosis of diabetic gastroparesis–a 25-year evaluation. Diabet Med 2013;30(5):e185–8.

Evaluation of Patients with Suspected Gastroparesis

Lawrence A. Szarka, MD, Michael Camilleri, MD*

KEYWORDS

- Gastric emptying • Functional dyspepsia • Rumination syndrome
- Cannabinoid hyperemesis • Opioids

KEY POINTS

- A careful history and physical examination should identify conditions known to be associated with gastroparesis and exclude mimics, such as rumination syndrome, cannabinoid hyperemesis, and drug-induced gastric emptying delay.
- Most patients will require focused laboratory testing, an anatomic evaluation with esophagogastroduodenoscopy or contrast radiography, and a validated measurement of gastric emptying.
- Functional disorders are much more common than gastroparesis. Patients who have normal or only mildly delayed gastric emptying should be diagnosed with functional dyspepsia.
- Patients with compromised nutritional status and moderate or severely delayed gastric emptying are appropriately diagnosed with gastroparesis.

INTRODUCTION

Gastroparesis, or paralysis of the stomach, implies that gastric emptying is delayed, despite the absence of any mechanical obstruction. Although this definition is straightforward, the diagnosis of gastroparesis is often inappropriately applied. Based on the authors' experience, many patients referred with the diagnosis of gastroparesis do not actually have this condition. The misdiagnosis is understandable because there is a limited repertoire of symptoms arising from the upper gastrointestinal (GI) tract, and there is overlap between the symptoms of gastroparesis and functional upper GI disorders. In general, gastroparesis is rare, with a community prevalence of 0.01%,[1]

Disclosure Statement: Dr M. Camilleri has research funding from Takeda for a study of TAK954 for gastroparesis. He has acted as a consultant to Ironwood, Takeda and Allergan regarding gastroparesis (with consulting fee going to his employer, Mayo Clinic). Dr L.A. Szarka has no conflicts of interest to disclose.
Division of Gastroenterology and Hepatology, Department of Medicine, Mayo Clinic College of Medicine and Science, Mayo Clinic, 200 First Street Southwest, Rochester, MN 55905, USA
* Corresponding author.
E-mail address: camilleri.michael@mayo.edu

functional disorders are far more prevalent,[2] and the results of the most important test to assess stomach function, gastric emptying scintigraphy (GES), needs to be interpreted with great caution.

Although gastroparesis can be acute due to infections such as norovirus, or due to metabolic conditions such as hyperglycemia, it is usually considered a chronic disease. Gastroparesis may be asymptomatic, as seen in some patients after gastric surgery who consistently have retained gastric contents on imaging.[3] However, the diagnosis of gastroparesis requires the presence of symptoms, not just objective delay in gastric emptying.

The cardinal symptoms associated with gastroparesis are nausea, vomiting, anorexia, early satiety, postprandial fullness, bloating, abdominal distention, and pain.[4,5] The severity of symptoms seems to be related to both levels of psychological distress and degree of gastric emptying delay.[6,7] The association of these symptoms with certain clinical scenarios, such as diabetes mellitus, previous gastric surgery, and connective tissue disorders, raises the possibility of gastroparesis. However, the most common attribution of gastroparesis is idiopathic, and the overwhelming majority of patients are women.[8] Although gastroparesis can be a devastating illness for some patients, most patients who have the diagnosis of gastroparesis do reasonably well, at least in terms of maintaining their hydration and nutritional status, which is ultimately the most important function of the GI system. Data from the National Institutes of Health Gastroparesis Clinical Research Consortium confirm that 45.7% of patients with gastroparesis have body mass index category of overweight or obese, and only 7.8% of patients are underweight.[6]

GENERAL APPROACH TO THE PATIENT WITH SUSPECTED GASTROPARESIS
History

Gastroparesis is suspected in patients who have the cardinal symptoms and also in patients who have the incidental finding of retained gastric contents on endoscopy or imaging studies performed for other indications (**Fig. 1**). Historical features that need to be queried include diabetes; connective tissue disorders, in particular scleroderma and Sjogren's syndrome, and any muscle symptoms suggestive of myopathy; and any thoracic or gastric surgeries that could have resulted in vagal injury, in particular fundoplication, and restrictive bariatric operations including laparoscopic adjustable gastric banding (**Box 1**).[9] Gastroparesis has also been reported after other procedures, including cardiac ablation for atrial fibrillation,[10] celiac plexus block,[11] and mesenteric revascularization.[12] Neurologic, specifically autonomic, symptoms such as anhidrosis or hyperhidrosis, orthostatism, sexual dysfunction, and bladder emptying problems should be elicited. A careful medication and drug use history needs to be obtained with regard to use of nonsteroidal anti-inflammatory drugs (NSAIDs) as a potential cause of dyspepsia and mechanical obstruction, opioids, anticholinergic medications, angiotensin-converting enzyme (ACE) inhibitors, and marijuana use (**Box 2**).

Careful attention should be paid to current symptoms, especially the description of vomiting, to distinguish true vomiting, which is characterized by association with intense nausea and forceful retching, from effortless postprandial regurgitation, which is highly suspicious for rumination syndrome. The patient's weight history needs to be carefully explored. As mentioned previously, only a small minority of patients with gastroparesis become underweight, but history of weight loss is a marker for severity. Self-reported weight, particularly for women, is unreliable,[13] and self-reporting of weight trends seems to be even more unreliable. When at all possible, documentation

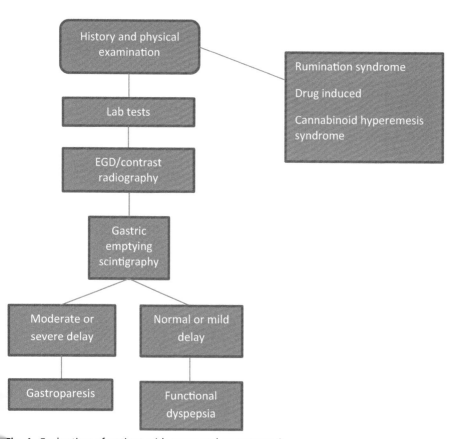

Fig. 1. Evaluation of patient with suspected gastroparesis.

of past weights in medical records should be found and recorded rather than accepting an unverified weight loss report.

The history should also explore lower GI symptoms, not just because their presence may signal an alternative diagnosis, such as irritable bowel syndrome, but also because constipation and rectal evacuation disorders may directly delay gastric emptying and cause the presenting upper GI symptomatology.[14–17] Finally, a psychiatric history has to be obtained with emphasis on eating disorders, anxiety, depression, and drug use, abuse, and neglect because psychiatric problems and undiagnosed eating disorders may masquerade as gastroparesis. Severe malnutrition, as seen in anorexia nervosa, can result in generalized slowing of physiologic functions, including gastric emptying, which typically resolves with regaining weight alone.[18]

Physical Examination

Height, weight, and vital sign documentation is necessary to assess current nutritional and hydration status, and provides a benchmark of progress over time. The patient's affect and appearance should be noted. Skin turgor, moistness of mucus membranes, and the presence or absence of axillary moisture provide additional information about hydration. Skin examination should also look for any rashes, tattoos of cannabis leaf, and features of scleroderma, such as microstomia, telangiectasias, and sclerodactyly.

Box 1
Selected causes of gastroparesis and delayed gastric emptying

Idiopathic

Diabetes mellitus

Postsurgery
  Antireflux
  Bariatric
  Distal gastrectomy
  Whipple procedure
  Heart or lung transplant

Connective tissue disorder
  Scleroderma
  Sjogren's
  Systemic lupus erythematosus
  Polymyositis/dermatomyositis

Amyloidosis

Anorexia nervosa

Autoimmune autonomic neuropathy

Chagas disease

Drug induced (see **Box 2**)

End-stage renal disease

Hollow visceral myopathy or neuropathy

Hypothyroidism

Malignancy
  Pancreas
  Lymphoma
  Paraneoplastic

Mesenteric ischemia

Neurologic disorders
  Parkinson disease
  Shy-Drager syndrome
  Muscular dystrophy
  Multiple sclerosis

The abdominal examination should include inspection for surgical scars and abdominal distention; auscultation for the presence or absence of bowel sounds (the complete absence of bowel sounds for 3 minutes indicates ileus, whereas the presence of louder high-pitched sounds with a tinkling quality suggest obstruction), vascular bruits, and the presence or absence of a succussion splash, which is elicited by rocking the patient back and forth at the hips or rapidly palpating the epigastrium. If abdominal tenderness to palpation is present, it should be noted if the patient has the closed eye sign or *la belle indifference* which is a feature of functional abdominal pain; the stethoscope sign indicates the diminishing of pain responses when palpating with the stethoscope in functional pain.[19] Palpation that reveals tenderness should also be repeated with abdominal wall tension maneuvers (ie, with straight legs raised) to distinguish visceral pain from myofascial pain, as may be expected in patients who have frequent retching, straining, and vomiting, or simply fibromyalgia.

Box 2
Selected medications that impair gastric emptying
Opioid analgesics

Anticholinergics
  Antipsychotics
  Antihistamines (first generation)
  Atropine
  Benztropine
  Dicyclomine
  Glycopyrrolate
  Hyoscyamine
  Oxybutynin
  Scopolamine
  Tricyclic antidepressants

Cannabinoids
  Dronabinol
  Tetrahydrocannabinol

Finally, a rectal examination should not be neglected merely because the patient is complaining of upper GI symptoms. As noted previously, rectal evacuation disorders can cause upper GI symptoms and impair gastric emptying, and many intractable GI problems are ultimately found to be due to inability to evacuate stool completely. Physical examination findings suggestive of rectal evacuation disorders include presence of high-resting anal tone, absence of perineal descent with straining, presence of stool in the rectum, and inadequate expulsive force or paradoxic sphincter contraction with simulated defecation.

Laboratory Testing

Initially, only basic laboratory tests are required, including complete blood count, glucose, electrolytes, blood urea nitrogen, creatinine, and thyroid-stimulating hormone. However, if a patient is diabetic, hemoglobin A1c testing is appropriate. If the patient is underweight or truly losing weight, then testing of cortisol (for Addison disease), nutritional markers, serum and urine protein, and immunoglobulin electrophoresis (for amyloidosis) should be performed. If there are physical signs of scleroderma, testing for the antinuclear antibodies, anti–scl-70 and anti-centromere, are reasonable. In patients with confirmed gastroparesis with unknown etiology who have evidence of extraintestinal autonomic dysfunction and personal or family history of other autoimmune diseases or substantial tobacco smoking history, testing for autoimmune gastrointestinal dysmotility with type 1 antineuronal nuclear and ganglionic nicotinic acetylcholine receptor autoantibodies and others[20,21] may also be appropriate. Rarely, testing for urinary and stool porphyrins, lead, and C-1 esterase inhibitor may be performed for unexplained abdominal pain and vomiting.[22] Finally, laboratory testing for over-the-counter, prescriptions and drug abuse screening are available and should be considered in view of surreptitious NSAID use and the opioid and cannabinoid consumption in the general population.[23]

CONDITIONS THAT MIMIC GASTROPARESIS

Even before undertaking any investigations, the pertinent historic elements can be revisited to diagnose or exclude the following conditions that may mimic gastroparesis; this often requires little or no additional investigation (**Box 3**).

Box 3
Gastroparesis mimics

Angiotensin-converting enzyme inhibitor–induced visceral angioedema

Anorexia nervosa

Antipsychotic-induced gastrointestinal dysmotility

Bulimia nervosa

Cannabinoid hyperemesis syndrome

Constipation due to rectal evacuation disorder

Cyclical vomiting syndrome

Functional dyspepsia

Functional nausea vomiting syndrome

Opioid-induced gastric emptying delay

Rumination syndrome

Rumination Syndrome

Diagnostic criteria for rumination syndrome consist of chronic effortless regurgitation (usually without nausea or retching) of recently ingested food into the mouth, with either spitting out or rechewing and reswallowing.[24] Rumination is recognized in all age groups; there is a female preponderance in children and adolescents,[25] and similar frequencies in both sexes in adulthood.[6] The regurgitation episode may be associated with an eructationlike or belchlike sensation. The mechanism appears to be a volitional increase in intra-abdominal pressure associated with simultaneous relaxations in the lower and upper esophageal sphincters.[26]

Regardless of the exact mechanism or whether the condition is gastric or supragastric,[27] recognition of typical symptoms of rumination obviates the need for extensive testing because the results can be misleading. For example, some patients with rumination syndrome have uninterpretable GES studies because they may regurgitate a large portion of the test meal before the first scintigraphic images are obtained. Another situation is that the gastric emptying may be slow because the regurgitation and reswallowing of food delays the delivery of the meal to the distal stomach for trituration. The treatment for rumination is behavior modification with habit reversal using diaphragmatic breathing exercises.[28,29]

Cyclical Vomiting and Cannabinoid Hyperemesis Syndromes

Cyclical vomiting syndrome (CVS) is characterized by discrete, stereotypical episodes of vomiting lasting less than 1 week and the absence of vomiting in-between episodes. Cannabinoid hyperemesis syndrome (CHS) is the presence of cyclical vomiting symptoms associated with prolonged, typically daily, marijuana use. Marijuana remains the most widely used illicit substance, with 13.2% of the population reporting use in 2014, and 3.5% reporting daily use.[30] Unlike patients with idiopathic gastroparesis, 88% of whom are female,[6] most adult patients with CVS are men and two-thirds of patients with CHS are men.[31] Patients with CVS and CHS typically have rapid or normal gastric emptying when studied between episodes.[32] The association between marijuana use and vomiting is said to be perplexing, but, more than 40 years ago, it was recognized that intravenous injection of cannabis infusion (tea) caused immediate abdominal pain and severe vomiting, leading to dehydration and renal failure.[33] Marijuana contains multiple cannabinoids that have pleiotropic effects. The best known cannabinoid, Δ9-tetrahydrocanabinol (THC), has central antiemetic action by binding to the cannabinoid receptor type 1 (CB1), but it retards gastric emptying at same dose,[34] whereas other cannabinoids are antagonists of CB1 or have biphasic responses with antiemetic activity at low doses, but emetogenic effects at higher doses.[35] Similarly, alcohol has a well-known spectrum of effects, ranging from excitation to depression, depending on the dose.

Opioid-Induced Gastroparesis

MOR (μ-opioid receptor) agonists cause a variety of GI motility abnormalities, including inhibition of antral contractility, augmentation of pyloric sphincter tone, increased fluid absorption and decreased propulsion in the small and large bowel, and increased anal sphincter tone.[36,37] These factors can delay gastric emptying, as demonstrated for example, with oxycodone (a selective MOR) and tapentadol (a combined MOR and norepinephrine reuptake inhibitor).[38] In addition to the peripheral effects, opioids can cause nausea and vomiting by central activation of the chemoreceptor trigger zone in the area postrema.[39]

The epidemiology of opioid use shows staggering numbers; based on the 2015 National Survey on Drug Use and Health, 37.8% of the adult population in the United States was prescribed opioids in 2015, and 4.7% misused opioids.[40] In a community survey conducted in Olmsted County, Minnesota, 4% of the population use opioids chronically.[41] It is inappropriate to perform GES on a patient taking opioids or withdrawing from them. It is equally confusing to appraise studies of gastroparesis in patients who are receiving or recently stopped opioids, because the neuronal effects of opioids may impact the presentation, natural history, and response to treatments.

Usual protocols for GES include recommendation to stop drugs that can impair motility for 72 hours, but this is not sufficient for long-acting opioids, such as methadone, which has a half-life up to 59 hours. In addition to the effective $T_{1/2}$, it is unknown how long neuronal plasticity induced by opioids actually persists and impairs neuromuscular function. The prevalence of opioid consumption in the population is such that drug testing should be considered before GES if there is any suspicion of surreptitious use.

Antipsychotic-Induced Dysmotility

Antipsychotic medications are increasingly common prescription drugs. The number of office visits resulting in a prescription for an antipsychotic nearly doubled from 1998 to 2002,[42] and the rates of prescribing second-generation antipsychotics (also known as atypical antipsychotics) and off-label use in children and adolescents have increased even more rapidly.[43] In general, the second generation of antipsychotics has greater anticholinergic activity than the first generation. Clozapine and olanzapine have exceptionally high binding affinities to peripheral muscarinic receptors.[44] Antipsychotic medication use is frequently associated with polypharmacy,[45] and the combination with other anticholinergic medications can result in severe dysmotility leading to frank pseudo-obstruction.[46] It is not appropriate to overlook this class of medication when performing GES or diagnosing anything other than drug-induced gastroparesis when the patient is exposed to these medications.

Angiotensin-Converting Enzyme Inhibitor–Related Visceral Angioedema

ACE inhibitors are among the most widely prescribed class of medications, with lisinopril being the most frequently prescribed of all drugs in the United States in

2017.[47] Angioedema as a side effect of ACE inhibitors occurs in 0.1% to 2.2% of people.[48] The onset of angioedema can occur anytime, even after many years of drug exposure.[49] ACE inhibitors are frequently prescribed to patients with diabetes to prevent progression of renal disease.

Gastrointestinal angioedema can cause episodes of obstructive symptoms of abdominal pain and vomiting. Radiographic findings of obstruction, bowel wall thickening, thumb printing, or ascites may be intermittent and, therefore, not apparent at the time of the radiological examination. There is no diagnostic test for ACE inhibitor–related angioedema, but patients with low alpha-1 antitrypsin levels are thought to be at increased risk. It is appropriate to consider the possibility of ACE inhibitor–induced visceral angioedema, especially in patients with diabetes who have otherwise unexplained episodes of vomiting. Use of a different class of antihypertensive medication with resolution of symptoms is required to confirm the diagnosis.

DIAGNOSTIC STUDIES
Upper Endoscopy

Esophagogastroduodenoscopy (EGD) is undoubtedly the most common test performed for the evaluation of upper GI symptoms and can assess for reflux esophagitis, gastritis (through gastric biopsy), peptic ulcer disease, pyloric stenosis, and visualize fasting gastric contents (bezoars, retained food, or excess bilious fluid). Bezoars are organized concretions of indigestible solids and are typically only seen in patients with postsurgical gastric atony. In contrast, the finding of some unorganized retained food is not uncommon at endoscopy and, therefore, should not be assumed to be diagnostic of gastroparesis. A recent review of factors associated with endoscopically identified gastric food retention by Coleski and colleagues[50] found that 24% of the evaluable patients had evidence of some luminal obstruction. Of the fraction of patients without obstruction who underwent GES, 74% were found to have delayed emptying, with the rates highest for patients with postsurgical gastroparesis, and the remainder had normal emptying. The finding of retained indigestible solids in the stomach after overnight fast and normal GES may be related to noncompliance with preprocedure fasting recommendations, or possibly due to the interindividual variability in the frequency of the migrating motor complex, which may occur as infrequently as just once daily in some healthy individuals.[51]

Concomitant opioid medication use was found in 40% of the patients with retained food. Conversely, only 27% of patients with delayed GES were found to have gastric retained food at endoscopy, with the highest rates for those with severe gastric emptying delays. Therefore, the finding of retained gastric contents mandates additional evaluation to exclude distal obstruction, opioid use, and gastroparesis. Only limited literature exists on the value of endoscopically observed antral contractility and pyloric motion, and its value in the assessment of gastroparesis remains unknown.[52]

Contrast Radiography

Contrast radiography with barium of the upper GI tract with small bowel follow-through is an alternative or complement to EGD. Contrast radiography will give a truer assessment of hiatal hernia because of the absence of gagging at intubation with the scope and the absence of gastric insufflation with gas (as long as effervescent agents are not added to the barium). Contrast radiography can assess not just immediate gastric outlet obstruction but also impingement by the superior mesenteric artery and more distal causes of small bowel obstruction. A carefully conducted barium study in patients with suggestive symptoms can frequently identify features that are suggestive of gastroparesis, including qualitatively decreased or absent peristalsis, dilated stomach, retained gastric contents, and qualitatively delayed gastric emptying of barium. The identification of the gastric dilation phenotype is rarely appreciated at endoscopy because it is always performed with gas insufflation.

On the other hand, barium is not a substitute for a formal gastric emptying test such as GES because barium is inert and lacks the physiochemical properties of food; it is hypo-osmolar compared with food. The interpretation of contrast studies is limited to stating when the first amount of barium emptied the stomach or when all of the barium emptied the stomach; it is not possible to say when a certain percentage, say 25% or 75%, of the barium left the stomach. Surprisingly, there are no normal values for how long it should take for barium to empty the stomach in healthy volunteers, although there are a few studies that have measured orocecal transit of barium in healthy volunteers.[53,54]

Gastric Emptying Scintigraphy

GES is considered the gold standard for the evaluation of how the stomach empties food and is the most commonly used method for the diagnosis of gastroparesis in the United States. There are 2 well-accepted GES protocols that define normal emptying rates at greater than or equal to 40% at 2 hours and greater than or equal to 90% at 4 hours with a 255-kcal (2% fat) meal; and greater than 25% at 2 hours and greater than 75% at 4 hours with a 320-kcal (30% fat) meal.[55] Consensus society guidelines for the performance of GES have been available for the past decade.[56] GES also provides stratification of severity (based on the 255-kcal, low-fat meal) as follows: mild (<90% to 80% emptying at 4 hours; or normal at 4 hours, but <40% emptying at 2 hours); moderate (<80% to 65% emptying at 4 hours); severe (<65% to 50% emptying at 4 hours); and very severe (<50% gastric emptying at 4 hours).[7] The 255-kcal meal has been criticized for not having enough fat, which is a well-known provocateur of symptoms in patients,[57] and perhaps neither meal is challenging enough to simulate normal eating patterns.

There is evidence (and lively debate) for and against the association of gastric emptying rates with symptoms, but what is clear is that, if a patient has a normal GES test, one can be confidant that a diet similarly composed would be appropriately handled by the patient's stomach and that they should not require heroic nutritional support.

Gastric Emptying Breath Test

The gastric-emptying breath test (GEBT) is a Food and Drug Administration (FDA)-approved, commercially available diagnostic kit that consists of a 238-kcal meal (41% fat) composed of ^{13}C-*Spirullina platensis* (a pharmaceutical grade, edible blue-green algae enriched with the stable 13-carbon isotope), scrambled egg, 6 saltine crackers, and 180 mL of water. After an 8-hour fast, breath samples are obtained for measurement of ratio of $^{13}CO_2/^{12}CO_2$ at baseline and at 45, 90, 120, 150, 180, and 240 minutes after ingestion of the test meal. The $^{13}CO_2$ and $^{12}CO_2$ in breath samples are stable and can be mailed to a central facility for analysis by mass spectrometry to determine the ratio of breath $^{12}CO_2/^{13}CO_2$. This ratio is used to calculate the metric called kPCD (percent dose excreted * 1000). The enrichment of breath with $^{13}CO_2$ is proportional to the gastric emptying rate. The $^{13}CO_2$ excretion rate versus time curve of the patient based on the sequential samples from baseline to 240 minutes is compared with the reference curve, which consists of time-specific lower limit cutoff points. Gastroparesis is diagnosed if the kPCD values are below the cutoff points at 90, 120, or 150 minutes, and the maximum excretion rate is shifted toward the 240-minute time point.

GEBT was well validated by studies using simultaneous GES of the same radiolabeled meal and demonstrates excellent performance characteristics.[58–60] The benefit of the GEBT is its ease of administration, so it can be performed anywhere and, significantly, it does not expose the patient to any radiation. The disadvantage is that it is not a direct assessment of gastric emptying because the $^{13}CO_2$ excretion rate also depends on the rate of intestinal digestion and absorption of the test meal components, and pulmonary gas exchange. Therefore, the test may be less reliable in patients with pancreatic insufficiency, malabsorption, and severe chronic obstructive pulmonary disease.

Wireless Motility Capsule

The wireless motility capsule (WMC) is also an FDA-approved device for the evaluation of gastric emptying. Similar to scintigraphy, but different from GEBT, the WMC can also assess small bowel and colonic transit. The WMC is an orally ingested, nondigestible capsule that measures temperature, pressure, and pH continuously, and transmits the information to a wearable external receiver. Characteristics of temperature and pH profile are used to determine the time of arrival into the stomach and the time of arrival into the small bowel to determine the gastric emptying time (GET).

The testing protocol to determine GET consists of discontinuation of acid suppressive medications (proton pump inhibitors 1 week before; and histamine-2 receptor antagonists for 3 days before), discontinuation of drugs affecting motility 3 days before, and avoidance of tobacco products and alcohol for 8 and 24 hours, respectively, before the test. After an overnight fast, a standard 260-kcal (2% fat) nutrient bar is ingested, followed immediately by the ingestion of the WMC. The patient must refrain from eating for the next 6 hours, and then may return to normal activity. A study of 87 healthy adults and 67 patients with gastroparesis undergoing simultaneous WMC and GES demonstrated correlation of 0.73 between GET measured by WMC and 4-hour scintigraphic emptying time.[61] However, this correlation included 29 (20%) of 148 data censored at the 6-hour value for gastric emptying time and also 10 participants (5 healthy controls and 5 patients) with WMC emptying time censored at 6 hours, whereas the scintigraphic measurement was completely normal with less than 10% retention at 4 hours.

The pitfall with WMC is that it is an indigestible solid and, therefore, it empties the stomach not with the test meal, but rather with the phase III activity front of the migrating motor complex. The return of the phase III activity front is a surrogate for the completion of gastric emptying of a nutritional meal. However, in some healthy individuals, a phase III–like activity front may be triggered within the first few minutes after meal ingestion, whereas other healthy individuals may have only one phase III during an entire day. Therefore, the GET determined by WMC may vary widely and may be quite different than the emptying of a nutritional meal from the stomach.[62]

Cross-Sectional Imaging

A final diagnostic consideration is for the subset of patients who are underweight or have documented weight loss and who have substantial upper abdominal pain. These patients should always have some cross-sectional imaging with either computed tomography or MRI to exclude pancreatic disease.

FUNCTIONAL DYSPEPSIA AND CHRONIC NAUSEA VOMITING SYNDROME VERSUS GASTROPARESIS

Functional upper GI disorders provide the most common cause of the misdiagnosis of gastroparesis. The Rome IV diagnostic criteria for chronic nausea vomiting syndrome (CNVS) are the presence of isolated nausea and/or vomiting at least 1 day per week for the past 3 months with the exclusion of self-induced vomiting, eating disorders, and rumination, in the absence of other diseases.[24] Functional dyspepsia (FD) is defined as chronic bothersome postprandial fullness and/or early satiation and/or epigastric pain and/or epigastric burning with the usual temporal and exclusionary criteria. FD is common, with prevalence between 10% and 30% in large studies.[63] CNVS is less common, occurring in just 2% to 3% of patients.[64] The symptoms of these 2 functional disorders completely overlap with the symptoms of gastroparesis, and virtually all patients with gastroparesis also meet criteria for FD. Indeed, approximately 25% to 35% of the patients with FD are reported to have some degree of delayed emptying.[65,66]

How then should the clinician distinguish FD with delayed emptying from a patient with gastroparesis? This must depend on 2 objective factors: first, the degree of gastric emptying delay and, second, the weight status of the patient. Considering that 5% of healthy subjects have gastric emptying values that are slower than the normal range by definition, it is not appropriate to have FD symptoms and only a mild gastric emptying delay to diagnose gastroparesis, which would expose the patient to a variety of treatments that have equivocal or unknown efficacy and definite potential for harm. Likewise, someone who is obese or overweight and has documented maintenance of weight on an oral diet should not be given a diagnosis of gastroparesis unless gastric emptying is profoundly delayed. It is also best to be cognizant that GI symptoms arise from both peripheral and central mechanisms, and the contribution of each varies in individual patients. It is more plausible that isolated gastric symptoms may arise from delayed gastric emptying, whereas the patient with wide ranging GI and extraintestinal functional disorders, psychiatric comorbidities, and extensive drug and food intolerances with a mild gastric emptying delay is unlikely to have the motility defect as the actual driver of their dyspepsia; that is, although the former patient may possibly have gastroparesis, the latter patient must be diagnosed with FD.

Finally, the symptoms of gastroparesis overlap with those of patients with either accelerated or delayed gastric emptying. Recent literature has also identified abnormalities of gastric accommodation that may occur alone or together with delayed gastric emptying in patients with the same spectrum or upper GI symptoms. In a 1287-patient cohort evaluated at Mayo Clinic over 15 years, approximately 25% had lone delay in gastric emptying, approximately 25% lone impaired gastric accommodation, and 25% combined delayed emptying and impaired gastric accommodation.[67] Gastric accommodation is best measured by invasive intragastric barostat balloon[68] or noninvasive single-photon emission computed tomography imaging.[69] Other "screening approaches" include a nutrient drink test with documentation of maximum tolerated volume,[70] intragastric pressure after food ingestion using high-resolution manometry,[71] measurement of the proximal stomach immediately after food ingestion in a GES study,[72] or MRI.[73]

SUMMARY

Although many patients have symptoms compatible with gastroparesis or a delayed gastric emptying problem, most of them have FD. Often times, the patients with the very worst symptoms have a drug-induced problem due to opioids, marijuana, atypical antipsychotics, or ACE inhibitors. The diagnosis of a drug-induced gastric symptom is critically important because it correctly implies that the only appropriate treatment will be drug cessation. The diagnosis of rumination syndrome can be made clinically without any additional diagnostic testing. Many other patients, however, will require laboratory tests to exclude metabolic problems, and possibly to identify the underlying cause of their gastroparesis. Most patients will need EGD and/or contrast radiography to exclude structural diseases. GES is still regarded as the gold standard to confirm the presence of gastric emptying delay and provides stratification of the severity of the motility impairment. In the absence of underweight status or documented weight loss, the patients with a mild degree of gastric emptying delay are best diagnosed as FD to protect them from inappropriate therapies. The remainder of the patients who have true gastroparesis can be considered for the treatments addressed in the rest of this issue.

REFERENCES

1. Jung HK, Choung RS, Locke GR 3rd, et al. The incidence, prevalence, and outcomes of patients with gastroparesis in Olmsted County, Minnesota, from 1996 to 2006. Gastroenterology 2009;136:1225–33.
2. Camilleri M, Dubois D, Coulie B, et al. Prevalence and socioeconomic impact of upper gastrointestinal disorders in the U.S.: results of the U.S. upper gastrointestinal study. Clin Gastroenterol Hepatol 2005;3:543–52.
3. Gonda TA, Woo Y. Miscellaneous diseases of the stomach. In: Podolsky DK, editor. Yamada's textbook of gastroenterology. 6th edition. Chichester (UK): John Wiley & Sons Ltd.; 2016. p. 1150–1.
4. Hasler WL, Wilson LA, Parkman HP, et al. Factors related to abdominal pain in gastroparesis: contrast to patients with predominant nausea and vomiting. Neurogastroenterol Motil 2013;25:427–38, e300–1.
5. Revicki DA, Rentz AM, Dubois D, et al. Development and validation of a patient-assessed gastroparesis symptom severity measure: the gastroparesis cardinal symptom index. Aliment Pharmacol Ther 2003;18:141–50.
6. Parkman HP, Yates K, Hasler WL, et al. Clinical features of idiopathic gastroparesis vary with sex, body mass, symptom onset, delay in gastric emptying, and gastroparesis severity. Gastroenterology 2011;140:101–15.
7. Hasler WL, Parkman HP, Wilson LA, et al. Psychological dysfunction is associated with symptom severity but not disease etiology or degree of gastric retention in patients with gastroparesis. Am J Gastroenterol 2010;105:2357–67.
8. Soykan I, Sivri B, Sarosiek I, et al. Demography, clinical characteristics, psychological and abuse profiles, treatment, and long-term follow-up of patients with gastroparesis. Dig Dis Sci 1998;43:2398–404.
9. Srikanth MS, Oh KH, Keskey T, et al. Critical extreme anterior slippage (paragastric Richter's hernia) of the stomach after laparoscopic adjustable gastric banding: early recognition and prevention of gastric strangulation. Obes Surg 2005;15:207–15.
10. Choi SW, Kang SH, Kwon OS, et al. A case of severe gastroparesis: indigestion and weight loss after catheter ablation of atrial fibrillation. Pacing Clin Electrophysiol 2012;35:e59–61.
11. Iftikhar S, Loftus EV Jr. Gastroparesis after celiac plexus block. Am J Gastroenterol 1998;93:2223–5.

12. Gauci JL, Stoven S, Szarka L, et al. Prolonged idiopathic gastric dilatation following revascularization for chronic mesenteric ischemia. Ann Gastroenterol 2014;27:273–5.
13. Merrill RM, Richardson JS. Validity of self-reported height, weight, and body mass index: findings from the National Health and Nutrition Examination Survey, 2001-2006. Prev Chronic Dis 2009;6:A121.
14. Shim L, Prott G, Hansen RD, et al. Prolonged balloon expulsion is predictive of abdominal distension in bloating. Am J Gastroenterol 2010;105:883–7.
15. Youle MS, Read NW. Effect of painless rectal distension on gastrointestinal transit of solid meal. Dig Dis Sci 1984;29:902–6.
16. Kellow JE, Gill RC, Wingate DL. Modulation of human upper gastrointestinal motility by rectal distension. Gut 1987;28:864–8.
17. Tjeerdsma HC, Smout AJPM, Akkermans LMA. Voluntary suppression of defecation delays gastric emptying. Dig Dis Sci 1993;38:832–6.
18. Rigaud D, Bedig G, Merrouche M, et al. Delayed gastric emptying in anorexia nervosa is improved by completion of a renutrition program. Dig Dis Sci 1988; 33:919–25.
19. Sperber AD, Drossman DA. Review article: the functional abdominal pain syndrome. Aliment Pharmacol Ther 2011;33:514–24.
20. Dhamija R, Tan KM, Pittock SJ, et al. Serologic profiles aiding the diagnosis of autoimmune gastrointestinal dysmotility. Clin Gastroenterol Hepatol 2008;6: 988–92.
21. Flanagan EP, Saito YA, Lennon VA, et al. Immunotherapy trial as diagnostic test in evaluating patients with presumed autoimmune gastrointestinal dysmotility. Neurogastroenterol Motil 2014;26:1285–97.
22. Beigel Y, Ostfeld I, Schoenfeld N. Clinical problem-solving. A leading question. N Engl J Med 1998;339:827–30.
23. Grant BF, Saha TD, Ruan WJ, et al. Epidemiology of DSM-5 drug use disorder: results from the national epidemiologic survey on alcohol and related conditions-III. JAMA Psychiatry 2016;73:39–47.
24. Talley NJ, Stanghellini V, Chan FKL, et al. Gastroduodenal disorders. In: Drossman DA, editor. Rome IV functional gastrointestinal disorders, vol. 2, 4th edition. Raleigh (NC): Rome Foundation; 2016. p. 903–65.
25. Chial HJ, Camilleri M, Williams DE, et al. Rumination syndrome in children and adolescents: diagnosis, treatment, and prognosis. Pediatrics 2003;111:158–62.
26. Rommel N, Tack J, Arts J, et al. Rumination or belching-regurgitation? Differential diagnosis using oesophageal impedance-manometry. Neurogastroenterol Motil 2010;22:e97–104.
27. Tucker E, Knowles K, Wright J, et al. Rumination variations: aetiology and classification of abnormal behavioural responses to digestive symptoms based on high-resolution manometry studies. Aliment Pharmacol Ther 2013;37:263–74.
28. Wagaman JR, Williams DE, Camilleri M. Behavioral intervention for the treatment of rumination. J Pediatr Gastroenterol Nutr 1998;27:596–8.
29. Halland M, Parthasarathy G, Bharucha AE, et al. Diaphragmatic breathing for rumination syndrome: efficacy and mechanisms of action. Neurogastroenterol Motil 2016;28:384–91.
30. Azofeifa A, Mattson ME, Schauer G, et al. National estimates of marijuana use and related indicators—national survey on drug use and health, United States, 2002-2014. MMWR Surveill Summ 2016;65:1–28.
31. Simonetto DA, Oxentenko AS, Herman ML, et al. Cannabinoid hyperemesis: a case series of 98 patients. Mayo Clin Proc 2012;87:114–9.

32. Hejazi RA, Lavenbarg TH, McCallum RW. Spectrum of gastric emptying patterns in adult patients with cyclic vomiting syndrome. Neurogastroenterol Motil 2010; 22:1298–302.e8.

33. Mims RB, Lee JH. Adverse effects of intravenous cannabis tea. J Natl Med Assoc 1977;69:491–5.

34. McCallum RW, Soykan I, Sridhar KR, et al. Delta-9-tetrahydrocannabinol delays the gastric emptying of solid food in humans: a double-blind, randomized study. Aliment Pharmacol Ther 1999;13:77–80.

35. Darmani NA. The potent emetogenic effects of the endocannabinoid, 2-AG (2-arachidonoylglycerol) are blocked by delta(9)-tetrahydrocannabinol and other cannnabinoids. J Pharmacol Exp Ther 2002;300:34–42.

36. Camilleri M, Malagelada JR, Stanghellini V, et al. Dose-related effects of synthetic human beta-endorphin and naloxone on fed gastrointestinal motility. Am J Physiol 1986;251(1 Pt 1):G147–54.

37. Musial F, Enck P, Kalveram KT, et al. The effect of loperamide on anorectal function in normal healthy men. J Clin Gastroenterol 1992;15:321–4.

38. Jeong ID, Camilleri M, Shin A, et al. A randomised, placebo-controlled trial comparing the effects of tapentadol and oxycodone on gastrointestinal and colonic transit in healthy humans. Aliment Pharmacol Ther 2012;35:1088–96.

39. Costello DJ, Borison HL. Naloxone antagonizes narcotic self blockade of emesis in the cat. J Pharmacol Exp Ther 1977;203:222–30.

40. Han B, Compton WM, Blanco C, et al. Prescription opioid use, misuse, and use disorders in U.S. adults: 2015 national survey on drug use and health. Ann Intern Med 2017;167:293–301.

41. Choung RS, Locke GR 3rd, Zinsmeister AR, et al. Opioid bowel dysfunction and narcotic bowel syndrome: a population-based study. Am J Gastroenterol 2009; 104:1199–204.

42. Aparasu RR, Bhatara V, Gupta S. U.S. national trends in the use of antipsychotics during office visits, 1998-2002. Ann Clin Psychiatry 2005;17:147–52.

43. Harrison JN, Cluxton-Keller F, Gross D. Antipsychotic medication prescribing trends in children and adolescents. J Pediatr Health Care 2012;26:139–45.

44. Chew ML, Mulsant BH, Pollock BG, et al. A model of anticholinergic activity of atypical antipsychotic medications. Schizophr Res 2006;88:63–72.

45. Correll CU, Gallego JA. Antipsychotic polypharmacy: a comprehensive evaluation of relevant correlates of a long-standing clinical practice. Psychiatr Clin North Am 2012;35:661–81.

46. Palmer SE, McLean RM, Ellis PM, et al. Life-threatening clozapine-induced gastrointestinal hypomotility: an analysis of 102 cases. J Clin Psychiatry 2008; 69:759–68.

47. Kane S. 2017 Top 200 drugs. ClinCalc DrugStats Database. 2017. Available at: http://clincalc.com. Accessed April 1, 2018.

48. Sánchez-Borges M, Capriles-Hulett A, Caballero-Fonseca F. NSAID-induced urticaria and angioedema: a reappraisal of its clinical management. Am J Clin Dermatol 2002;3:599–607.

49. Malde B, Regalado J, Greenberger PA. Investigation of angioedema associated with the use of angiotensin-converting enzyme inhibitors and angiotensin receptor blockers. Ann Allergy Asthma Immunol 2007;98:57–63.

50. Coleski R, Baker JR, Hasler WL. Endoscopic gastric food retention in relation to scintigraphic gastric emptying delays and clinical factors. Dig Dis Sci 2016;61: 2593–601.

51. Wilson P, Perdikis G, Hinder RA, et al. Prolonged ambulatory antroduodenal manometry in humans. Am J Gastroenterol 1994;89:1489–95.

52. Niwa H, Nakamura T, Fujino M. Endoscopic observation on gastric peristalsis and pyloric movement. Gastroenterological Endoscopy 1975;17:236–42.

53. Lönnerblad L. Transit time through small intestine: roentgenologic study on normal variability. Acta Radiol Suppl 1951;88:1–85.

54. Thompson WM, Halvorsen RA, Shaw M, et al. Evaluation of intramuscular ceruletide for shortening small bowel transit time. Gastrointest Radiol 1982;7:141–7.

55. Pasricha PJ, Camilleri M, Hasler WL, et al. White Paper AGA: gastroparesis: clinical and regulatory insights for clinical trials. Clin Gastroenterol Hepatol 2017;15:1184–90.

56. Abell TL, Camilleri M, Donohoe K, et al. Consensus recommendations for gastric emptying scintigraphy: a joint report of the American Neurogastroenterology and Motility Society and the Society of Nuclear Medicine. Am J Gastroenterol 2008;103:753–63.

57. Feinle-Bisset C, Azpiroz F. Dietary and lifestyle factors in functional dyspepsia. Nat Rev Gastroenterol Hepatol 2013;10:150–157.3.

58. Szarka LA, Camilleri M, Vella A, et al. A stable isotope breath test with a standard meal for abnormal gastric emptying of solids in the clinic and in research. Clin Gastroenterol Hepatol 2008;6:635–43.e1.

59. Odunsi ST, Camilleri M, Szarka LA, et al. Optimizing analysis of stable isotope breath tests to estimate gastric emptying of solids. Neurogastroenterol Motil 2009;21:706-e38.

60. Bharucha AE, Camilleri M, Veil E, et al. Comprehensive assessment of gastric emptying with a stable isotope breath test. Neurogastroenterol Motil 2013;25:e60–9.

61. Kuo B, McCallum RW, Koch KL, et al. Comparison of gastric emptying of a non-digestible capsule to a radio-labelled meal in healthy and gastroparetic subjects. Aliment Pharmacol Ther 2008;27:186–96.

62. Szarka LA, Camilleri M. Methods for measurement of gastric motility. Am J Physiol Gastrointest Liver Physiol 2009;296:G461–75.

63. Mahadeva S, Goh KL. Epidemiology of functional dyspepsia: a global perspective. World J Gastroenterol 2006;12:2661–6.

64. Talley NJ, Ruff K, Jiang X, et al. The Rome III classification of dyspepsia: will it help research? Dig Dis 2008;26:203–9.

65. Tack J, Lee KJ. Pathophysiology and treatment of functional dyspepsia. J Clin Gastroenterol 2005;39(5 Suppl 3):S211–6.

66. Perri F, Clemente R, Festa V, et al. Patterns of symptoms in functional dyspepsia: role of *Helicobacter pylori* infection and delayed gastric emptying. Am J Gastroenterol 1998;93:2082–8.

67. Park SY, Acosta A, Camilleri M, et al. Gastric motor dysfunction in patients with functional gastroduodenal symptoms. Am J Gastroenterol 2017;112:1689–99.

68. Sarnelli G, Vos R, Cuomo R, et al. Reproducibility of gastric barostat studies in healthy controls and in dyspeptic patients. Am J Gastroenterol 2001;96:1047–53.

69. Bouras EP, Delgado-Aros S, Camilleri M, et al. SPECT imaging of the stomach: comparison with barostat, and effects of sex, age, body mass index, and fundoplication. Single photon emission computed tomography. Gut 2002;51:781–6.

70. Tack J, Caenepeel P, Piessevaux H, et al. Assessment of meal induced gastric accommodation by a satiety drinking test in health and in severe functional dyspepsia. Gut 2003;52:1271–7.

71. Janssen P, Verschueren S, Ly HG, et al. Intragastric pressure during food intake: a physiological and minimally invasive method to assess gastric accommodation. Neurogastroenterol Motil 2011;23:316–22.
72. Orthey P, Yu D, Van Natta ML, et al. Intragastric meal distribution during gastric emptying scintigraphy for assessment of fundic accommodation: correlation with symptoms of gastroparesis. J Nucl Med 2018;59(4):691–7.
73. Fidler J, Bharucha AE, Camilleri M, et al. Application of magnetic resonance imaging to measure fasting and postprandial volumes in humans. Neurogastroenterol Motil 2009;21:42–51.

Symptomatic Management of Gastroparesis

Christopher M. Navas, MD[a],*, Nihal K. Patel, MD[b], Brian E. Lacy, MD, PhD[c]

KEYWORDS

- Abdominal pain • Antiemetics • Diabetes • Gastroparesis • Nausea • Vomiting

KEY POINTS

- The most frequently reported symptoms of gastroparesis are those of nausea, vomiting, epigastric pain, early satiety, and weight loss.
- Treatment for gastroparesis should be individualized and focus on the most bothersome symptom, which varies from patient to patient.
- Although delayed gastric emptying is, by definition, a unifying finding in all patients with gastroparesis, accelerating or normalizing gastric emptying may not improve symptoms.
- A variety of medications are available to treat symptoms of nausea and vomiting, although metoclopramide remains the only medication approved by the Food and Drug Administration for gastroparesis.
- Epigastric pain, reported by up to 90% of patients with gastroparesis, can be treated with a number of different anti-nociceptive agents, although opioids should not be prescribed.

INTRODUCTION

Gastroparesis is a chronic, bothersome and often disabling neuromuscular disorder of the upper gastrointestinal tract. Gastroparesis, defined as delayed gastric emptying in the absence of mechanical obstruction, can be accurately diagnosed using a combination of subjective symptoms and objective measures[1] (see Lawrence A. Szarka and Michael Camilleri's article, "Evaluation of Patients with Suspected Gastroparesis," in this issue). The most commonly reported symptoms of gastroparesis include nausea, vomiting, early satiety, abdominal pain, bloating and weight loss (**Box 1**). Unfortunately, these symptoms are nonspecific and cannot be used to accurately diagnose

Disclosure Statement: None of the authors have any commercial or financial conflicts for this article.
[a] Department of Internal Medicine, Dartmouth-Hitchcock Medical Center, 1 Medical Center Drive, Lebanon, NH 03756, USA; [b] Section of Gastroenterology and Hepatology, Dartmouth-Hitchcock Medical Center, 1 Medical Center Drive, Lebanon, NH 03756, USA; [c] Division of Gastroenterology and Hepatology, Mayo Clinic, 4500 San Pablo Road, Jacksonville, FL 32224, USA
* Corresponding author. PO Box 969, Quechee, VT 05059.
E-mail address: Christopher.m.navas@hitchcock.org

Gastrointest Endoscopy Clin N Am 29 (2019) 55–70
https://doi.org/10.1016/j.giec.2018.08.005
1052-5157/19/© 2018 Elsevier Inc. All rights reserved.

Box 1
Common symptoms of gastroparesis

Nausea: 90% to 95%

Epigastric pain: 89% to 90%

Early satiety: 80% to 85%

Vomiting: 65%

Bloating

Gastroesophageal reflux disease

Anorexia

Weight loss

---

gastroparesis nor distinguish gastroparesis from other disorders of gastric neuromuscular dysfunction, such as functional dyspepsia.[2] In addition, individual symptoms do not accurately predict the extent of delayed gastric emptying.[1,3–8] This article briefly reviews and defines the most common symptoms reported by patients with gastroparesis, and then evaluates therapeutic options for each symptom.

Nausea is present in nearly all patients with gastroparesis.[1,3,4] Derived from the Greek word *nautia* (seasickness), nausea is defined as a vague, unpleasant feeling of unease with the sensation that vomiting might occur. Nausea is a subjective feeling and is difficult to objectively measure. Anorexia frequently precedes the onset of nausea, whereas objective symptoms of pallor, hypersalivation, diaphoresis, and tachycardia are common. Vomiting is reported by at least two-thirds of patients with gastroparesis.[3,4] In the evaluation of patients with suspected gastroparesis, it is important to carefully distinguish vomiting from regurgitation and rumination. Vomiting is characterized by the forceful ejection of gastric contents from the mouth. Regurgitation, a cardinal symptom of gastroesophageal reflux disease, is characterized by the effortless and involuntary movement of gastric contents into the mouth without abdominal wall contractions.[9] Rumination is a voluntary process in which patients effortlessly bring up recently ingested food from the stomach into the mouth, where it is then chewed again and reswallowed.[10] In contrast to patients with gastroparesis, nausea, pallor, hypersalivation and tachycardia are not seen in patients with rumination. Early satiety is a sensation of being overly full after eating a normal or modest-sized meal.[11] It is present in 80% to 85% of patients with gastroparesis.[1,4] Early satiety is also a cardinal symptom of functional dyspepsia and can be present in patients with delayed gastric emptying but also in those with normal gastric emptying, but impaired gastric accommodation or abnormal visceral sensation.[12] Bloating is commonly reported by patients with gastroparesis. Bloating, or a sensation of gassiness, should be distinguished from distension, which involves a change in abdominal girth.[13] Although not formally studied in large populations, the etiology of bloating in patients with gastroparesis, like that of functional dyspepsia and irritable bowel syndrome (IBS), is likely varied and diverse and includes disordered visceral hypersensitivity, alterations in the gut microbiome, small intestinal bacterial overgrowth, and carbohydrate intolerance. Up to 90% of patients with gastroparesis report symptoms of epigastric pain.[5] The pain is considered functional in nature, as the definition of gastroparesis suggests that an organic cause for symptom generation and expression cannot be identified on upper endoscopy.[1,3] Finally, some patients with gastroparesis suffer from weight loss. As an isolated symptom, weight loss is nonspecific, as it is commonly found in other functional gastrointestinal disorders, including patients with functional dyspepsia and normal gastric emptying.[11] However, patients with unintentional weight loss greater than 10% of ideal body weight should be assessed for possible nutritional compromise. In the following section, therapeutic agents for each symptom are reviewed.

NAUSEA AND VOMITING

In patients with gastroparesis, nausea and vomiting are multifactorial symptoms arising from impaired gastric fundus tone, antral hypomotility, antroduodenal dyscoordination, dysrhythmias of the gastric pacemaker, and excessive inhibitory feedback from the small bowel.[14] Nausea and vomiting are complex processes orchestrated by a collection of nuclei located in the dorsal lateral reticular formation of the medulla referred to as the central vomiting center. Afferent signals are transmitted to the central vomiting center from the back of the throat, gastrointestinal tract, vestibular system, and the chemoreceptor trigger zone (CTZ) (a bundle of neurons located in the area postrema). This pathway of neurons responds to both noxious stimuli and gastrointestinal irritants through various receptors. Control of these symptoms in clinical practice relies on the use of one medication approved by the Food and Drug Administration (FDA) (metoclopramide) and off-label use of antiemetic medications that have demonstrated efficacy in chemotherapy-induced or postoperative nausea and vomiting (PONV) (**Table 1**).

Metoclopramide is a centrally acting dopamine D_2-receptor antagonist and remains the only FDA-approved medication for the treatment of gastroparesis symptoms. Metoclopramide exhibits antiemetic effects via inhibition of D_2 and $5-HT_3$ receptors in the brain, as well as prokinetic effects as a $5-HT_4$ receptor agonist in the gut.[15] Metoclopramide can be administered through multiple routes, although the oral solution is the preferred way to improve absorption. Clinical guidelines recommend starting at the lowest possible effective dose for each patient beginning with 5 mg 3 times a day 30 minutes before meals with a maximum dose of 40 mg/d.[1] The use of metoclopramide is often limited by undesired side effects ranging from mild sedation and agitation, to extrapyramidal effects. Metoclopramide carries a black box warning

Table 1
Suggested medications for symptoms of nausea and vomiting in gastroparesis

Medications	Oral Dose
Metoclopramide	5–10 mg 3 to 4 times a day
Domperidone[b]	10 mg 3 to 4 times a day
Ondansetron[a]	8 mg 3 times a day
Prochlorperazine[a]	5–10 mg 4 times a day
Chlorpromazine[a]	10–25 mg 4 times a day
Scopolamine[a]	1.5 mg patch every 3 d
Aprepitant[a]	80 mg every day
Dronabinol[a]	5–10 mg 3 times a day
Tricyclic antidepressants[a]	25–100 mg/d
Ginger	1 g twice a day

Off-label use.
Only available for use in the United States via Food and Drug Administration investigational drug protocol.

restricting its use to $\leq$12 weeks for the risk of tardive dyskinesia, although this risk is believed to be small (<1%).[16]

Domperidone, a dopamine D_2-receptor antagonist, is similar in action to metoclopramide, although it is peripherally acting and does not readily cross the blood brain barrier.[17] It is associated with fewer central side effects. There is an association of domperidone with QT prolongation and ventricular tachycardia.[18] Domperidone is available in the United States only through an FDA investigational drug application. The recommended starting dosage is 10 mg 3 times a day with escalation to 20 mg 4 times a day including bedtime.[1] A recent single-center cohort study (n = 115) of patients with gastroparesis showed that most (68%) patients treated with domperidone had improvement in symptom scores. This study also noted that 7% (8 of 115) of patients had cardiac-type side effects necessitating stopping.[19]

5-HT$_3$ receptor antagonists and phenothiazines are commonly used off-label for the treatment of nausea and vomiting of gastroparesis. 5-HT$_3$ receptor antagonists inhibit vagal afferent nerves, as well as receptors in the chemoreceptor trigger zone but do not affect gastrointestinal motility.[20,21] All first-generation 5-HT$_3$ antagonists have similar efficacy, and therefore selection can be determined by price and availability.[22] Ondansetron is available in both parenteral and enteral forms, including an oral disintegrating tablet, whereas granisetron is now available in a transdermal delivery system. In 2 studies, transdermal granisetron (3.1 mg/24 h) was effective in decreasing symptom scores by 50% in patients with refractory gastroparesis symptoms.[23,24] Phenothiazines (eg, prochlorperazine and chlorpromazine) inhibit D_1 and D_2 receptors in the brain leading to antiemetic effects. There have not been any studies directly comparing 5-HT$_3$ receptor agonists and phenothiazines.[1]

A variety of other medications are available to treat nausea and vomiting but the data behind their use in gastroparesis is limited. Scopolamine is a muscarinic cholinergic receptor antagonist that has been used off-label for the treatment of nausea in patients with gastroparesis, although there have not been any clinical studies to support its use.[1] Aprepitant is an NK-1 receptor antagonist that reduces nausea and vomiting through the inhibition of substance P in the area postrema.[25,26] A recent randomized control trial of 126 patients with gastroparesis treated with aprepitant (125 mg/d, n = 63) observed mixed results, as it failed to demonstrate a reduction in visual analog scores but did show reduction in Gastroparesis Cardinal Symptom Index (GCSI) scores.[27] Further studies are needed to assess its use in gastroparesis. Tricyclic antidepressants (TCAs; described later in this article) can be considered in patients with gastroparesis with refractory nausea and vomiting.[1] Synthetic cannabinoids (eg, dronabinol, nabilone) are approved for the treatment of nausea and vomiting associated with chemotherapy, but their use in gastroparesis has not yet been formally evaluated. Cannabinoids have the potential to slow gastric emptying, which may worsen some gastroparesis symptoms.

Patients often explore complementary and alternative medicines for relief of symptoms. Although the exact antiemetic mechanism of ginger extract is unclear, it may inhibit serotonin receptors in the gut.[28] A meta-analysis of 5 randomized trials (n = 363) demonstrated that a dose of 1 g of ginger was more effective than placebo for the prevention of PONV.[28] Acupuncture is used in a variety of diseases, although its efficacy for gastroparesis symptoms remains unclear. The results from a meta-analysis of acupuncture in patients with gastroparesis were inconclusive given the low quality of trials/studies included in the analysis.[29] Relaxation techniques including guided imagery and hypnosis have shown in several research studies to be helpful in alleviating nausea and vomiting in patients undergoing chemotherapy.[30]

ABDOMINAL PAIN

Although gastroparesis is recognized by the classic symptoms of nausea, vomiting, early satiety, and postprandial fullness, abdominal pain is a frequent symptom that may be overlooked and requires special attention.[5] Various studies have reported a prevalence of abdominal pain in 46% to 89% of patients with gastroparesis. A questionnaire-based study of 68 patients reported a similar prevalence in both diabetic and idiopathic patients with gastroparesis.[31] Pain was commonly located in the epigastrium (42%); present daily in 43% of patients, most often induced by eating (72%), and frequently nocturnal, interfering with sleep (66% of patients). The severity of abdominal pain was reported as comparable to other gastroparetic symptoms, such as nausea and vomiting, and correlated significantly with impaired quality of life.[31]

Unfortunately, the pathophysiology of abdominal pain in gastroparesis is poorly understood. Delayed gastric emptying has not been proven to be a causative factor.[32] The overlapping nature of pain symptoms in gastroparesis and functional dyspepsia suggests that similar pathophysiological mechanisms, such as a hypersensitivity to gastric distention or an impaired accommodation of the stomach fundus to meals, are likely responsible.[33,34] In diabetic patients with gastroparesis, autonomic neuropathy could play a role in pain symptoms; however, one small study reported that severe forms of visceral afferent neuropathy were associated with fewer, rather than greater, symptoms.[35] To date, there have not been any large randomized studies to address the efficacy of any therapy specifically for the management of abdominal pain in patients with gastroparesis. The following section reviews data on medications that are frequently used by clinicians (**Table 2**), with evidence extrapolated from trials in functional dyspepsia, IBS, and diabetic polyneuropathy.

Many clinicians initiate treatment for gastroparetic patients with mild pain with an antispasmodic medication, such as dicyclomine or hyoscyamine.[36] Although not studied in patients with gastroparesis, these medications have been used extensively to treat abdominal pain in IBS. Benefits are thought to occur via their anticholinergic effects, resulting in intestinal smooth muscle relaxation. Similarly, peppermint oil capsules or tea may also be considered for the treatment of mild symptoms.[37]

Table 2
Suggested medications for management of abdominal pain

Name	Class	Recommended Dose
Dicyclomine	Anticholinergic	20 mg 4 times a day as needed
Hyoscyamine	Anticholinergic	0.125–0.25 mg 3 to 4 times a day as needed
Amitriptyline	TCA	25–100 mg/d
Desipramine	TCA	25–75 mg/d
Mirtazapine	Antidepressant	7.5–30 mg/d
Duloxetine	SNRI	60–120 mg/d
Gabapentin	Anticonvulsant	>1200 mg/d in divided doses
Pregabalin	Anticonvulsant	100–300 mg/d in divided doses
Tapentadol	μ-opioid agonist	Start at 50 mg twice a day
Tramadol	μ-opioid agonist	200 mg/d in divided doses

Abbreviations: SNRI, serotonin and norepinephrine reuptake inhibitors; TCA, tricyclic antidepressant.

For more bothersome symptoms, visceral neuromodulatory medications should be considered. These agents reduce the perception of pain and act at different levels of the brain-gut axis via multiple mechanisms. One of the main targets for these treatments is serotonin (5-HT), the predominant neurotransmitters in the enteric nervous system.[38]

TCAs (eg, amitriptyline, desipramine, nortriptyline) have been extensively used in clinical practice to modulate pain. In low doses, these medications may also decrease symptoms of nausea and vomiting. Possible side effects include dry mouth, dry eyes, and urinary retention. One placebo-controlled, randomized trial has evaluated a TCA in gastroparesis. The NORIG trial[39] studied the effect of nortriptyline, dose-escalated at 3-week intervals up to 75 mg at 12 weeks, on overall symptoms of idiopathic gastroparesis in 130 patients. Using a strict primary outcome of greater than or equal to 50% reduction in overall GCSI scores on 2 consecutive assessments compared with the baseline, this study showed no difference between the nortriptyline group and placebo. There was also no significant difference in abdominal pain subscores between both groups. This study raises doubts regarding the efficacy of nortriptyline particularly in patients with idiopathic gastroparesis. Nevertheless, given multiple studies indicating positive results in the treatment of functional dyspepsia and its efficacy noted in clinical experience with other functional bowel disorders, TCAs should still be considered as an option to treat pain related to gastroparesis.

Selective serotonin reuptake inhibitors (SSRIs) enhance the effects of 5-HT by prolonging the availability of this neurotransmitter at neural synapses in both the central and enteral nervous systems. SNRIs (serotonin and norepinephrine reuptake inhibitors) work by blocking the reuptake of both serotonin and norepinephrine in a similar fashion. Various SSRIs and SNRIs, such as venlafaxine, sertraline, and escitalopram, have been studied in large well-designed clinical trials in patients with functional dyspepsia, yet have shown no benefit over placebo.[40] The SSRI paroxetine has been shown to enhance gastric accommodation and accelerate small intestinal transit in healthy adults,[38,41] but there are no data to support its use in patients with bowel disorders. Mirtazapine is an antidepressant with noradrenergic and specific serotonergic activity shown in multiple case reports as being effective for refractory nausea and vomiting.[42] A recent trial in patients with functional dyspepsia indicated that it was effective in reducing symptoms of dyspepsia and depression, and resulted in a significant increase in body weight.[43] A therapeutic trial of mirtazapine is a reasonable option in patients with gastroparesis with abdominal pain, who may also have refractory nausea and vomiting with weight loss. Buspirone is a selective serotonin 5-HT 1A partial agonist that relaxes the proximal stomach in healthy individuals, with a small clinical trial reporting significant improvements in the overall severity of symptoms of dyspepsia and a reduction in individual symptoms of postprandial fullness, early satiety, and upper abdominal bloating.[44] This same study indicated, however, that gastric emptying of liquids was delayed in patients treated with buspirone compared with placebo and evidence supporting its role in management of pain related to gastroparesis is lacking. It is an option if alternate therapies are unsuccessful.

Multiple medications have been shown to be effective for the treatment of diabetic polyneuropathy. These should be considered in the management of pain related to gastroparesis because it may be proposed that both conditions follow a similar pathophysiology. Duloxetine, for example, has been shown to result in significant improvements in diabetic polyneuropathic pain in 3 randomized placebo-controlled trials involving 1102 subjects, with both 60 and 120 mg daily over 12 weeks, compared with placebo. The side effects reported included nausea, somnolence, dizziness, decreased appetite, or constipation.[45-47] Evidence for venlafaxine in the treatment of painful diabetic neuropathy, on the other hand, has been less compelling based on a large systematic review of 6 randomized controlled trials with 460 patients.[48] Moreover, topiramate, an antiepileptic drug studied for the treatment of neuropathic pain, has shown no evidence of efficacy in patients with diabetic neuropathic pain based on a systematic review with data from 3 randomized trials and is thus not recommended.[49]

Gabapentin and pregabalin are other options for patients with gastroparesis pain. Gabapentin is frequently used for the management of neuropathic pain and a systematic review provided second-tier evidence that patients achieving at least a >50% reduction in pain was higher in patients on gabapentin dosed at greater than 1200 mg daily in divided doses, compared with placebo.[50] Unfortunately, some of the evidence supporting this efficacy has been called into question due to selective outcome reporting by industry-sponsored trials for off-label use.[51] Pregabalin binds to a subunit of the voltage-gated calcium channels within the central nervous system and modulates calcium influx, inhibiting release of excitatory neurotransmitters and exerting antinociceptive and anticonvulsant effects. It is structurally related to gabapentin but has no activity at GABA or benzodiazepine receptors. Pooled analysis from 7 randomized clinical trials enrolling 1510 patients over 5 to 13 weeks indicated a statistically significant reduction in mean pain score at treatment doses of 150 mg, 300 mg, and 600 mg daily over divided doses. Common reported side effects included dizziness, somnolence, weight gain, and peripheral edema.[52]

Opioid analgesics (eg, morphine, oxycodone, hydromorphone) should not be used to manage chronic visceral abdominal pain, as they further delay gastric emptying, increase the risk of narcotic bowel syndrome, and create the potential for addiction, tolerance, and overdose. If absolutely required, the weak μ-opioid agonist, tramadol, which also acts as an SNRI, could be considered at the lowest effective dose, although it does significantly delay colon transit in healthy patients and there are no data of efficacy available in patients with gastroparesis.[1] In patients with diabetic neuropathy, an average dose of 210 mg/d was more effective than placebo.[53] Alternatively, a medication called tapentadol can be used, which is a related compound with both μ-opioid agonism (with a lower affinity compared with classic opioids) and norepinephrine reuptake inhibition. Trials in patients with painful diabetic neuropathy reported that extended release tapentadol at 100 to 250 mg twice daily resulted in a statistically significant improvement in pain compared with placebo. Side effects reported included nausea, diarrhea, anxiety, constipation, and dizziness.[54]

Although data supporting the use of the previously mentioned medications specifically in patients with gastroparesis are lacking, therapeutic trials of at least 8 weeks with each drug should be considered with monitoring for clinical improvement. A suggested order for treatment of moderate to severe pain includes TCA, duloxetine, pregabalin or gabapentin, tramadol or tapentadol, along with consideration of supplemental therapies such as Iberogast or cognitive behavioral therapy (mentioned elsewhere).

EARLY SATIETY

Early satiety is present in 80% to 85% of patients with gastroparesis[1,4] and is described as not being able to finish a normal sized meal due to a sense of fullness. The pathophysiology of early satiety is secondary to abnormal proximal gastric function including impaired accommodation and delayed gastric emptying.[55] Treatment is often difficult, as there are limited options currently available. Symptom relief usually involves dietary changes such as eating smaller, more frequent meals and the use of prokinetic medications.

Metoclopramide and domperidone (as described previously) act as prokinetic agents by blocking dopamine in the gut leading to increased gastric tone, improvement in intragastric pressure and increased antroduodenal coordination.[56] Metoclopramide is also a moderate 5-HT$_4$ agonist contributing to its prokinetic effects.[25] 5-HT$_4$ receptor agonists are potent prokinetic agents that stimulate the peristaltic reflex through release of acetylcholine at the myenteric plexus.[25,57] Unfortunately, drugs of this class (cisapride and tegaserod) have been removed from the market due to undesired cardiac adverse effects. Velusetrag is a highly selective 5-HT$_4$ receptor agonist currently undergoing clinical trials. In healthy subjects, velusetrag has shown acceleration of gastric emptying halftime after consecutive daily doses, without cardiac side effects.[58] Prucalopride is another selective 5-HT$_4$ receptor agonist that has shown improvement in both gastric emptying halftime and GCSI scores in idiopathic patients with gastroparesis.[59] However, prucalopride is not currently available for use in the United States.

Erythromycin is a macrolide antibiotic that acts as a motilin receptor agonist and is commonly used off-label in gastroparesis. Activation of motilin receptors in the gastrointestinal tract stimulate cholinergic activity in the antrum and initiation of phase III contractions of the migrating motor complex (MMC)[60-62] helping move material from the stomach to the intestines. Hospitalized patients can be treated with erythromycin IV (over 45 minutes) at a dosage of 3 mg/kg every 8 hours.[1] For outpatients, oral doses of 50 to 100 mg 4 times a day given 30 to 45 minutes before each of the 3 main meals and at bedtime may improve symptoms.[14] Unfortunately, after weeks of continued use, most patients develop tachyphylaxis to erythromycin, limiting its effectiveness. Camicinal, a motilin receptor agonist currently in clinical trials, has shown to improve gastric emptying times in diabetic patients with gastroparesis without a decrease in response after 28 days of use.[63] Ghrelin is an endogenous peptide that is also involved in stimulation of phase III of the MMC.[64] Relamorelin is a potent synthetic ghrelin agonist currently in clinical trials. It has been shown to improve gastric emptying halftime and GCSI scores in diabetic patients with gastroparesis.[65,66]

Other potential treatments for early satiety in gastroparesis include acotiamide and STW 5 (Iberogast). Acotiamide acts as both a muscarinic antagonist and an acetylcholinesterase inhibitor.[67] Muscarinic receptor antagonists increase acetylcholine levels leading to prokinetic effects through antral contractility.[68] Acotiamide has been shown to significantly accelerate gastric emptying halftime, increase gastric accommodation, and improve early satiety in patients with functional dyspepsia,[55,69] but no studies have been performed using patients with gastroparesis. STW 5 (Iberogast) is a combination product (containing 9 herbal extracts) reported to improve upper abdominal symptoms in functional dyspepsia. STW 5 is believed to enhance antral motility and relaxation of the proximal stomach,[70] but does not appear to have an effect on gastric emptying.[71] It has been shown to be superior to placebo in improving symptom scores in 3 randomized controlled studies of patients with functional dyspepsia.[68] Although STW 5 has not been tested in trials using patients with gastroparesis, it was noted that patients with dysmotility-like dyspepsia had a greater decrease in symptom scores with STW 5.[71]

BLOATING

Bloating is a commonly encountered complaint by patients in all fields of medicine. Although more than 90% of patients with IBS report bloating, this symptom is also highly prevalent in patients with gastroparesis.[72] The etiology for bloating is not well understood, but potential mechanisms include visceral hypersensitivity, alterations in gut microflora, and changes in intestinal gas production or transit. There also may be impaired mechanisms of gas evacuation and an abnormal abdominal-diaphragmatic reflex resulting in physical distention, which accompanies, but is distinct from the sensation of bloating.[73] Multiple studies have also indicated a high prevalence rate of small intestinal bacterial overgrowth ranging from 39% to 60% in patients with gastroparesis, which likely also plays a role.[74,75]

Treatment can be difficult. There are no randomized clinical trials with improvement in bloating as a primary outcome when evaluating therapeutic options in patients with gastroparesis. Recommendations (**Box 2**) are based on studies performed in patients with IBS or based on expert clinical opinion. The initial step in management of bloating involves recognizing the symptom, educating the patient about the potential pathophysiology, and then reassuring the patient that these symptoms, although bothersome and frustrating, are not life-threatening.

A simple initial intervention may be the recommendation that the patient change his or her diet. Avoiding foods that ferment easily in the colon, more specifically avoiding FODMAP (fermentable oligo-, di-, mono-saccharides and polyols) food products has been shown to improve bloating symptoms in patients with IBS. Furthermore, although there are no large well-designed studies to support this, patients may report improvement in symptoms after avoiding fiber, or after minimizing carbohydrates and gluten. Avoiding carbonated drinks and food additives that cause excessive gas production, along with increased physical exercise, also may help.[72]

Altering gut flora is postulated to help improve symptoms. This may be achieved by the use of probiotics, which have been shown to improve bloating symptoms in patients with IBS. Specifically, 2 studies have shown that patients randomized to *Bifidobacterium infantis* 35624 experienced improved symptoms of bloating. VSL #3, which contains 450 billion bacteria per capsule and is a mixture of multiple strains of bacteria, has also been shown in few small studies to result in improved symptoms of bloating compared with placebo.[72]

Antibiotics have been well studied for the treatment of bloating. The most studied is rifaximin, a poorly absorbable gut selective antibiotic. Based on 2 large placebo-controlled studies with 1260 nonconstipated patients with IBS (TARGET 1 and TARGET 2 studies), patients treated with rifaximin 550 mg 3 times daily for 2 weeks had significant relief of bloating compared with patients receiving placebo.[76]

Prokinetics have been discussed in detail elsewhere in this article. In brief, domperidone may improve symptoms of bloating although there have been no randomized

---

Box 2
Suggested interventions for the management of bloating

Dietary changes (low FODMAP [fermentable oligo-, di-, mono-saccharides and polyols] diet, avoidance of fiber or gluten and minimizing carbohydrates)

Probiotics (*Bifidobacterium infantis* 35624 or VSL#3)

Poorly absorbable antibiotics such as rifaximin (550 mg 3 times a day for 2 weeks)

Pain neuromodulators, such as tricyclic antidepressants or pregabalin

Polyethylene glycol or calcium channel activators (linaclotide 145–290 µg daily) to improve slow transit

Hypnotherapy

trials evaluating its efficacy. One small study involving metoclopramide indicated that it did not improve symptoms of abdominal distention in patients with dyspepsia.[77] Neostigmine, used in the hospital setting, has been shown to result in immediate clearance of retained gas; however, a small placebo-controlled study using pyridostigmine in patients with IBS with bloating showed only a slight improvement in bloating symptoms.[78]

Medications used to treat chronic idiopathic constipation have a role in the treatment of bloating in gastroparesis. The use of polyethylene glycol has been shown to improve symptoms of bloating in patients with chronic constipation. The calcium channel activator, linaclotide, taken once daily at 145 and 290 μg, has been shown to significantly improve symptoms of bloating compared with placebo in patients with chronic idiopathic constipation.[73] Finally, hypnotherapy has been consistently shown to reduce symptoms of bloating in patients with IBS and can be considered in gastroparesis as well.[79]

WEIGHT LOSS

Unintentional weight loss is reported by many, but not all, patients with gastroparesis. In fact, some patients with documented gastroparesis are obese. The exact prevalence of weight loss in patients with gastroparesis is not known, in part because resolution of weight loss has not been either a primary or secondary endpoint in any large therapeutic trial of patients with gastroparesis. As well, when recorded, weight loss is usually reported as an absolute number (eg, pounds or kilograms), rather than as a percentage of ideal body weight. The precise etiology of weight loss in patients with gastroparesis is unknown, and likely varies based on the underlying cause (eg, postinfectious vs diabetic vs postsurgical). In some patients, weight loss may be related to pain that develops after eating, whereas in others, fear of developing postprandial nausea and vomiting may limit oral intake. Prospective trials with well-defined endpoints are required to resolve these issues.

A variety of therapeutic options are available to help patients with gastroparesis regain lost weight. However, because resolution of weight loss has not been a defined endpoint in any large gastroparesis trial to date, the therapies listed in the following paragraphs are reviewed based on clinical experience and data from other conditions associated with weight loss, some of which are gastrointestinal in origin (eg, functional dyspepsia), whereas others are nongastrointestinal in origin (eg, cancer). Of note, none of the agents discussed are approved by the FDA specifically for the treatment of weight loss in patients with gastroparesis, and thus technically all use would be considered off-label.

The first step to assist patients with gastroparesis with regaining lost weight is to take a detailed dietary history. The patient should track daily calorie counts for at least 1 week. Laboratory studies should be performed to determine whether the patient is nutritionally compromised; a body mass index should be calculated and used as a reference point. Referral to a dietician may be appropriate. For many patients, small changes in diet or eating behavior may be all that is required. These changes may include the following: minimizing water intake and instead substituting liquids with calories; drinking nutritional supplements; removing low-calorie foods and substituting in calorie-dense foods; and eating smaller, but more frequent meals. One prospective study found that diabetic patients with gastroparesis improved with a small particle-size diet.[80]

The second step is to identify and treat the most bothersome symptom. For example, persistent nausea or postprandial nausea may lead to weight loss, and ant-emetic therapy may be all that is required. In other patients, treating the pain associated with gastroparesis may lead to an improvement in weight. Some agents used to treat neuropathic pain are associated with weight gain when used to treat other conditions (eg, TCAs). Other patients with gastroparesis may lose weight due to a conditioned response. When eating predictably causes pain or nausea or vomiting, some patients restrict oral intake. Medical therapies combined with cognitive behavioral therapy may be required in patients who have developed a food aversion.

If weight loss fails to improve with the steps outlined previously, then additional medical therapy may be required (**Table 3**). It is important to note that none of these agents has been studied prospectively in patients with gastroparesis using randomized, placebo-controlled trials. In addition, it is worth noting that the addition of these medications to other medications that the patient may already be taking creates the potential for polypharmacy and the potential for adverse effects. Thus, a careful discussion with the patient outlining the benefits, risks, and costs of the medication is essential.

TCAs (mentioned previously) have been safely used for years to treat neuropathic pain in many diverse painful conditions (eg, diabetic neuropathy, fibromyalgia, shingles). Patients should be started on a low dose and then the TCA should slowly be titrated upward, balancing the potential benefits of weight gain with possible side effects. Use of a low-dose TCA at bedtime may be particularly effective in patients with concomitant insomnia.

SSRIs are now one of the most frequently prescribed class of medications, primarily for the treatment of depression and anxiety. Although most SSRIs are not associated with weight gain, paroxetine (Paxil) has been reported to cause unintentional weight gain in many patients. It is not known if the weight gain is directly related to changes in serotonin uptake. This side effect can be used to a therapeutic advantage to help some patients with gastroparesis gain weight, especially if they have c-existing anxiety or depression.

Cyproheptadine (Periactin) is an older, and frequently forgotten, medication used to treat pediatric and adolescent patients with functional dyspepsia and functional abdominal pain. It acts as both an antihistamine and a serotonin antagonist. A starting dose of 4 mg per day is recommended and this can be titrated up to 4 mg 3 times a day. The most common side effects are those associated with antihistamines (dry mouth, dry eyes, urinary retention). Quetiapine (Seroquel) is classified as an atypical antipsychotic and is generally prescribed for patients with depression, bipolar disorder, and insomnia. Although not routinely used by most gastroenterologists, this

Table 3
Medications that may help patients with gastroparesis gain weight

Name	Class	Recommended Dose
Amitriptyline	TCA	25–100 mg/d
Desipramine	TCA	25–75 mg/d
Paroxetine	SSRI	20–40 mg/d
Cyproheptadine	Antihistamine	4 mg 3 times a day
Quetiapine	Antipsychotic	200–400 mg/d
Mirtazapine	Antidepressant	7.5–30 mg/d

Abbreviations: SSRI, selective serotonin reuptake inhibitor; TCA, tricyclic antidepressant.

can be useful for patients who have failed other therapies. As it may cause sedation in some patients, we generally recommend prescribing the medication for evening use, starting at a low dosage of 25 mg each night, and then titrating upward as necessary. Mirtazapine (Remeron) is a tetracyclic antidepressant and acts as a noradrenergic antagonist. It is most commonly used to treat depression, although it is also used to treat insomnia. Patients should be started on a low dosage (7.5 mg each evening) and monitored carefully, as some patients note side effects of worsening nausea or new-onset anxiety. Megestrol acetate (Megace), a progestational agent, is an older medication used as an orexigenic in patients with cancer or AIDS. It has not been studied specifically in patients with gastroparesis. Dosages as high as 240 to 800 mg/d are reported in the oncology literature, although because it has not been tested in patients with gastroparesis, we recommend that therapeutic trials start at a much lower dosage of 40 mg per day, with slow titration upward. Last, medical marijuana appears to be a logical choice for patients with gastroparesis with persistent weight loss who have failed other therapies. Although intrinsically appealing due to reported improvements in symptoms of nausea and vomiting in some patients, marijuana has the potential to worsen gastroparesis symptoms due to binding to endogenous cannabinoid receptors, resulting in a slowing of gastric emptying. This theoretic concern, and the very real potential to cause hyperemesis cannabis syndrome, dampens enthusiasm for the use of marijuana to help patients with gastroparesis gain weight.

SUMMARY

Gastroparesis affects approximately 5 to 10 million adult Americans (see Baha Moshiree and colleagues' article, "Epidemiology and Pathophysiology of Gastroparesis," in this issue). For many patients, symptoms are, unfortunately, chronic in nature and often disabling. The persistent symptoms of pain, nausea, and vomiting reduce a patient's quality of life and impose a significant negative economic impact to the health care system.[81] Unfortunately, gastroparesis can be difficult to treat, because patients typically present with multiple nonspecific symptoms, individual symptoms do not predict response to therapy, and medications designed to accelerate gastric emptying may not lead to symptom improvement. Unfortunately, no biomarkers have been identified that predict therapeutic response. Finally, treatment choices can be difficult, because a validated treatment algorithm does not exist, and the field of gastroparesis lacks head-to-head studies comparing different therapeutic agents. Treatment for patients with gastroparesis should be individualized and should focus on the most bothersome symptom. For patients with gastroparesis with mild symptoms, dietary changes and antiemetics used on an as-needed basis may be all that is required. Patients with persistent symptoms will require more intensive therapy, often using 1 or 2 antiemetics routinely, ensuring that symptoms of abdominal pain are addressed as well. For those who fail adequate trials of medical therapy, novel endoscopic treatments for gastroparesis are now available, recognizing that some of these therapies have not been subjected to validation in large, randomized, placebo-controlled trials. Fortunately, a renewed interest in this field has stimulated both regulatory agencies and pharmaceutical companies to look for innovative solutions that should improve symptoms of gastroparesis in the years to come.

REFERENCES

1. Camilleri M, Parkman HP, Shafi MA, et al. Clinical guideline: management of gastroparesis. Am J Gastroenterol 2013;108:18–37.

2. Lacy BE. Functional dyspepsia and gastroparesis: one disease or two? Am J Gastroenterol 2012;107:1615–20.
3. Parkman HP, Hasler WL, Fisher RS, et al, for the American Gastroenterological Association. American Gastroenterological Association medical position statement: diagnosis and treatment of gastroparesis. Gastroenterology 2004;127: 1589–91.
4. Soykan I, Sivri B, Sarosiek I, et al. Demography, clinical characteristics, psychological and abuse profiles, treatment, and long-term follow-up of patients with gastroparesis. Dig Dis Sci 1998;43:2398–404.
5. Hoogerwerf WA, Pasricha PJ, Kalloo AN, et al. Pain: the overlooked symptom in gastroparesis. Am J Gastroenterol 1999;94:1029–33.
6. Keshavarzian A, Iber FL, Vaeth J. Gastric emptying in patients with insulin-requiring diabetic mellitus. Am J Gastroenterol 1987;82:29–35.
7. Horowitz M, Maddox AF, Wishart JM, et al. Relationships between oesophageal transit and solid and liquid gastric emptying in diabetes mellitus. Eur J Nucl Med 1991;18:229–34.
8. Jones KL, Russo A, Stevens JE, et al. Predictors of delayed gastric emptying in diabetes. Diabetes Care 2001;24:1264–9.
9. Lacy BE, Weiser K, Chertoff J, et al. The diagnosis of gastroesophageal reflux disease. Am J Med 2010;123:583–92.
10. Absah I, Rishi A, Talley NJ, et al. Rumination syndrome: pathophysiology, diagnosis and treatment. Neurogastroenterol Motil 2017;29. https://doi.org/10.1111/nmo.12954.
11. Stanghellini V, Chan FKL, Hasler WL, et al. Gastroduodenal disorders. Gastroenterology 2016;150:1380–92.
12. Vanheel H, Carbone F, Valvekens L, et al. Pathophysiologic abnormalities in functional dyspepsia subgroups according to the Rome III criteria. Am J Gastroenterol 2017;112:132–40.
13. Malegelada JR, Accarino A, Azpiroz F. Bloating and abdominal distension: old misconceptions and current knowledge. Am J Gastroenterol 2017;112:1221–31.
14. Lacy BE, Weiser K. Gastric motility, gastroparesis, and gastric stimulation. Surg Clin North Am 2005;85(5):967–87.
15. Perkel MS, Moore C, Hersh T, et al. Metoclopramide therapy in patients with delayed gastric emptying. Dig Dis Sci 1979;24(9):662–6.
16. Rao AS, Camilleri M. Metoclopramide and tardive dyskinesia. Aliment Pharmacol Ther 2010;31(1):11–9.
17. Barone JA. Domperidone: a peripherally acting dopamine2-receptor antagonist. Ann Pharmacother 1999;33(4):429–40.
18. Drolet B, Rousseau G, Daleau P, et al. Domperidone should not be considered a no-risk alternative to cisapride in the treatment of gastrointestinal motility disorders. Circulation 2000;102(16):1883–5.
19. Schey R, Saadi M, Midani D, et al. Domperidone to treat symptoms of gastroparesis: benefits and side effects from a large single-center cohort. Dig Dis Sci 2016;61(12):3545–51.
20. Hasler WL. Serotonin and the GI tract. Curr Gastroenterol Rep 2009;11(5): 383–91.
21. Youssef AS, Parkman HP, Nagar S. Drug-drug interactions in pharmacologic management of gastroparesis. Neurogastroenterol Motil 2015;27(11):1528–41.
22. Navari R, Gandara D, Hesketh P, et al. Comparative clinical trial of granisetron and ondansetron in the prophylaxis of cisplatin-induced emesis. The Granisetron Study Group. J Clin Oncol 1995;13(5):1242–8.

23. Simmons K, Parkman HP. Granisetron transdermal system improves refractory nausea and vomiting in gastroparesis. Dig Dis Sci 2014;59(6):1231–4.
24. Midani D, Parkman HP. Granisetron transdermal system for treatment of symptoms of gastroparesis: a prescription registry study. J Neurogastroenterol Motil 2016;22(4):650.
25. Dumitrascu DL, Weinbeck M. Domperidone versus metoclopramide in the treatment of diabetic gastroparesis. Am J Gastroenterol 2000;95(1):316.
26. Hesketh PJ, Grunberg SM, Gralla RJ, et al. The oral neurokinin-1 antagonist aprepitant for the prevention of chemotherapy-induced nausea and vomiting: a multinational, randomized, double-blind, placebo-controlled trial in patients receiving high-dose cisplatin—the Aprepitant Protocol 052 Study Group. J Clin Oncol 2003; 21(22):4112–9.
27. Pasricha PJ, Yates KP, Sarosiek I, et al. Aprepitant has mixed effects on nausea and reduces other symptoms in patients with gastroparesis and related disorders. Gastroenterology 2018;154(1):65–76.e11.
28. Chaiyakunapruk N, Kitikannakorn N, Nathisuwan S, et al. The efficacy of ginger for the prevention of postoperative nausea and vomiting: a meta-analysis. Am J Obstet Gynecol 2006;194(1):95–9.
29. Yang M, Li X, Liu S, et al. Meta-analysis of acupuncture for relieving non-organic dyspeptic symptoms suggestive of diabetic gastroparesis. BMC Complement Altern Med 2013;13(1):311.
30. Rhodes VA, McDaniel RW. Nausea, vomiting, and retching: complex problems in palliative care. CA Cancer J Clin 2001;51(4):232–48.
31. Cherian D, Sachdeva P, Fisher RS, et al. Abdominal pain is a frequent symptom of gastroparesis. Clin Gastroenterol Hepatol 2010;8(8):676–81.
32. Hasler WL, Wilson LA, Parkman HP, et al. Factors related to abdominal pain in gastroparesis: contrast to patients with predominant nausea and vomiting. Neurogastroenterol Motil 2013;25(5):427.
33. Anaparthy R, Pehlivanov N, Grady J, et al. Gastroparesis and gastroparesis-like syndrome: response to therapy and its predictors. Dig Dis Sci 2009;54(5): 1003–10.
34. Karamanolis G, Caenepeel P, Arts J, et al. Association of the predominant symptom with clinical characteristics and pathophysiological mechanisms in functional dyspepsia. Gastroenterology 2006;130(2):296–303.
35. Rathmann W, Enck P, Frieling T, et al. Visceral afferent neuropathy in diabetic gastroparesis. Diabetes Care 1991;14(11):1086–9.
36. Brandt LJ, Chey WD, Foxx-Orenstein AE, et al. An evidence-based systematic review on the management of irritable bowel syndrome. Am J Gastroenterol 2009; 104(Suppl 1):S1–35.
37. Cappello G, Spezzaferro M, Grossi L, et al. Peppermint oil (Mintoil®) in the treatment of irritable bowel syndrome: a prospective double blind placebo-controlled randomized trial. Dig Liver Dis 2007;39(6):530–6.
38. Tack J, Sarnelli G. Serotonergic modulation of visceral sensation: upper gastrointestinal tract. Gut 2002;51(suppl 1):i77–80.
39. Parkman HP, Van Natta ML, Abell TL, et al. Effect of nortriptyline on symptoms of idiopathic gastroparesis: the NORIG randomized clinical trial. JAMA 2013;310: 2640–9.
40. Talley NJ, Ford AC. Functional dyspepsia. N Engl J Med 2015;373(19):1853–63.
41. Chial HJ, Camilleri M, Burton D, et al. Selective effects of serotonergic psychoactive agents on gastrointestinal functions in health. Am J Physiol Gastrointest Liver Physiol 2003;284(1):G130–7.

42. Hasler WL. Symptomatic management for gastroparesis: antiemetics, analgesics, and symptom modulators. Gastroenterol Clin North Am 2015;44(1):113–26.
43. Jiang SM, Jia L, Liu J, et al. Beneficial effects of antidepressant mirtazapine in functional dyspepsia patients with weight loss. World J Gastroenterol 2016; 22(22):5260.
44. Tack J, Janssen P, Masaoka T, et al. Efficacy of buspirone, a fundus-relaxing drug, in patients with functional dyspepsia. Clin Gastroenterol Hepatol 2012; 10(11):1239–45.
45. Goldstein DJ, Lu Y, Detke MJ, et al. Duloxetine vs. placebo in patients with painful diabetic neuropathy. Pain 2005;116(1–2):109–18.
46. Raskin J, Pritchett YL, Wang F, et al. A double-blind, randomized multicenter trial comparing duloxetine with placebo in the management of diabetic peripheral neuropathic pain. Pain Med 2005;6(5):346–56.
47. Wernicke JF, Pritchett YL, D'souza DN, et al. A randomized controlled trial of duloxetine in diabetic peripheral neuropathic pain. Neurology 2006;67(8):1411–20.
48. Gallagher HC, Gallagher RM, Butler M, et al. Venlafaxine for neuropathic pain in adults. Cochrane Database Syst Rev 2015;8:CD011091.
49. Wiffen PJ, Derry S, Lunn MP, et al. Topiramate for neuropathic pain and fibromyalgia in adults. Cochrane Database Syst Rev 2013;(8):CD008314.
50. Freeman R, Durso-DeCruz E, Emir B. Efficacy, safety, and tolerability of pregabalin treatment for painful diabetic peripheral neuropathy: findings from seven randomized, controlled trials across a range of doses. Diabetes care 2008;31(7):1448–54.
51. Vedula SS, Bero L, Scherer RW, et al. Outcome reporting in industry-sponsored trials of gabapentin for off-label use. N Engl J Med 2009;361(20):1963–71.
52. Moore RA, Wiffen PJ, Derry S, et al. Gabapentin for chronic neuropathic pain and fibromyalgia in adults. Cochrane Database Syst Rev 2011;(3):CD007938.
53. Harati Y, Gooch C, Swenson M, et al. Double-blind randomized trial of tramadol for the treatment of the pain of diabetic neuropathy. Neurology 1998;50(6):1842–6.
54. Schwartz S, Etropolski M, Shapiro DY, et al. Safety and efficacy of tapentadol ER in patients with painful diabetic peripheral neuropathy: results of a randomized-withdrawal, placebo-controlled trial. Curr Med Res Opin 2011;27(1):151–62.
55. Nakamura K, Tomita T, Oshima T, et al. A double-blind placebo controlled study of acotiamide hydrochloride for efficacy on gastrointestinal motility of patients with functional dyspepsia. J Gastroenterol 2017;52(5):602–10.
56. Tonini M, Cipollina L, Poluzzi E, et al. Clinical implications of enteric and central D2 receptor blockade by antidopaminergic gastrointestinal prokinetics. Aliment Pharmacol Ther 2004;19(4):379–90.
57. Briejer MR, Akkermans LM, Schuurkes JA. Gastrointestinal prokinetic benzamides: the pharmacology underlying stimulation of motility. Pharmacol Rev 1995;47(4):631–51.
58. Manini ML, Camilleri M, Goldberg M, et al. Effects of Velusetrag (TD-5108) on gastrointestinal transit and bowel function in health and pharmacokinetics in health and constipation. Neurogastroenterol Motil 2010;22(1):42.
59. Carbone F, Rotondo A, Andrews CN, et al. 1077 a controlled cross-over trial shows benefit of prucalopride for symptom control and gastric emptying enhancement in idiopathic gastroparesis. Gastroenterology 2016;150(4):S213–4.
60. Sarna SK. Cyclic motor activity; migrating motor complex. Gastroenterology 1985;89:894–913.
61. Broad J, Mukherjee S, Samadi M, et al. Regional- and agonist-dependent facilitation of human neurogastrointestinal functions by motilin receptor agonists. Br J Pharmacol 2012;167:763–74.

62. Sanger GJ, Furness JB. Ghrelin and motilin receptors as drug targets for gastro-intestinal disorders. Nat Rev Gastroenterol Hepatol 2016;13(1):38–48.

63. Barton ME, Otiker T, Johnson LV, et al. A randomized, doubleblind, placebo-controlled phase II study (MOT114479) to evaluate the safety and efficacy and dose response of 28 days of orally administered camicinal in diabetics with gastroparesis. Gastroenterology 2014;146:S-20.

64. Tack J, Depoortere I, Bisschops R, et al. Influence of ghrelin on interdigestive gastrointestinal motility in humans. Gut 2006;55:327–33.

65. Lembo A, Camilleri M, McCallum R, et al. Relamorelin reduces vomiting frequency and severity and accelerates gastric emptying in adults with diabetic gastroparesis. Gastroenterology 2016;151:87–96.

66. Camilleri M, McCallum RW, Tack JF, et al. Relamorelin in patients with diabetic gastroparesis: efficacy and safety results from a phase 2b randomized, double-blind, placebo-controlled, 12-week study (RM-131-009). Gastroenterology 2017;152(5):S139–40.

67. Lacy BE, Talley NJ, Locke G3, et al. Current treatment options and management of functional dyspepsia. Aliment Pharmacol Ther 2012;36(1):3–15.

68. Parkman HP, Trate DM, Knight LC, et al. Cholinergic effects on human gastric motility. Gut 1999;45(3):346–54.

69. Matsueda K, Hongo M, Tack J, et al. A placebo-controlled trial of acotiamide for meal-related symptoms of functional dyspepsia. Gut 2012;61(6):821–8.

70. Pilichiewicz AN, Horowitz M, Russo A, et al. Effects of Iberogast® on proximal gastric volume, antropyloroduodenal motility and gastric emptying in healthy men. Am J Gastroenterol 2007;102(6):1276.

71. Braden B, Caspary W, Börner N, et al. Clinical effects of STW 5 (Iberogast®) are not based on acceleration of gastric emptying in patients with functional dyspepsia and gastroparesis. Neurogastroenterol Motil 2009;21(6):632.

72. Lacy BE, Gabbard SL, Crowell MD. Pathophysiology, evaluation, and treatment of bloating: hope, hype, or hot air? Gastroenterol Hepatol 2011;7(11):729.

73. Lacy BE, Schey R, Shiff SJ, et al. Linaclotide in chronic idiopathic constipation patients with moderate to severe abdominal bloating: a randomized, controlled trial. PLoS One 2015;10(7):e0134349.

74. George NS, Sankineni A, Parkman HP. Small intestinal bacterial overgrowth in gastroparesis. Dig Dis Sci 2014;59(3):645–52.

75. Reddymasu SC, McCallum RW. Small intestinal bacterial overgrowth in gastroparesis: are there any predictors? J Clin Gastroenterol 2010;44(1):e8–13.

76. Pimentel M, Lembo A, Chey WD, et al. Rifaximin therapy for patients with irritable bowel syndrome without constipation. N Engl J Med 2011;364(1):22–32.

77. Accarino A, Perez F, Azpiroz F, et al. Intestinal gas and bloating: effect of prokinetic stimulation. Am J Gastroenterol 2008;103(8):2036.

78. Johnson AG. Controlled trial of metoclopramide in the treatment of flatulent dyspepsia. Br Med J 1971;2(5752):25–6.

79. Agrawal A, Houghton LA, Lea R, et al. Bloating and distention in irritable bowel syndrome: the role of visceral sensation. Gastroenterology 2008;134(7):1882–9.

80. Olausson EA, Störsrud S, Grundin H, et al. A small particle size diet reduces upper gastrointestinal symptoms in patients with diabetic gastroparesis: a randomized controlled trial. Am J Gastroenterol 2014;109:375–85.

81. Lacy BE, Crowell MD, Mathis C, et al. Gastroparesis: quality of life and healthcare utilization. J Clin Gastroenterol 2018;52(1):20–4.

Gastric Electrical Stimulator for Treatment of Gastroparesis

Hadi Atassi, DO[a], Thomas L. Abell, MD[b],*

KEYWORDS

• Gastric electrical stimulation • Gastroparesis • Enterra

KEY POINTS

- Gastric electrical stimulation has been shown to provide symptomatic improvement to those suffering from gastroparesis that is refractory to conservative management.
- Temporary gastric electrical stimulation can be used in patients to determine if they will have a positive response to a permanent gastric electrical stimulator.
- Pyloric therapy is an alternative option for those who do not have a positive response to gastric electrical stimulation or whose symptoms worsen after gastric electrical stimulation.
- Some patients may have neuromuscular abnormalities, making them refractory to gastric stimulation but amenable to immunotherapy.

INTRODUCTION

Gastroparesis is a syndrome of delayed gastric emptying in which patients experience a variety of symptoms, including nausea, vomiting, abdominal pain, and early satiety. This delayed gastric emptying can be due to abnormal myoelectrical activity or abnormal gastric motility, with 2 common causes being diabetes mellitus and prior gastric surgery with vagotomy. Treatment options have evolved over the years. Initial management consists of dietary modifications, glycemic control, and pharmacologic therapy, typically metoclopramide or erythromycin, as well as nutritional

Disclosure Statement: Dr T.L. Abell has been an investigator for Medtronic, Rhythm, Theravance, Vanda, and Allergan, and a consultant for Theravance. He is the GI Section Editor for Med Study, GI Stimulation editor for *Neuromodulation*, GES editor for Wikistim, and a reviewer for UpToDate. Dr T.L. Abell is the founder of ADEPT-GI, which holds intellectual property covering some aspects of technology in this article. There are no other disclosures.
[a] Department of Medicine, Division of Internal Medicine, University of Louisville, 550 South Jackson Street, ACB A3K00, Louisville, KY 40202, USA; [b] Department of Medicine, Division of Gastroenterology, Hepatology and Nutrition, University of Louisville, 550 South Jackson Street, ACB A3L15, Louisville, KY 40202, USA
* Corresponding author.
E-mail address: thomas.abell@louisville.edu

Gastrointest Endoscopy Clin N Am 29 (2019) 71–83
https://doi.org/10.1016/j.giec.2018.08.013
1052-5157/19/© 2018 Elsevier Inc. All rights reserved.

supplementation, either through enteral or parenteral feedings. Unfortunately, around 30% of patients fail conservative management.[1] This failure of therapy results in frequent hospitalizations and a worsened quality of life. As such, when patient's symptoms fail to be controlled with said management, the next step is to consider implantation of a gastric electrical stimulator (GES) for medically refractory gastroparesis. Over time, studies have shown that a GES can decrease symptoms in patients with medically refractory gastroparesis.[1] This article aims to look at the use of GES in patients with gastroparesis as well as some of the new advances in therapy. However, not all patients benefit from GES; pyloric myotomy is a new strategy currently being studied that has shown promising results for those patients.

BACKGROUND

The idea of using GES was predicated on the knowledge that the human gastrointestinal tract is made up of natural pacemakers, like that of our coronary system. The stomach consists of a series of electrical potentials, termed slow waves, that span from the greater curvature of the stomach (where the pacemaker is placed) all the way along the greater wall toward the pylorus.[2] Propagation of slow waves toward the pylorus typically occurs every 20 seconds, so about 3 cycles per minute. The pylorus itself lacks slow-wave activity and essentially acts as a barrier between the cells in the duodenum and those of the stomach.[3] The slow waves originate in the interstitial cells of Cajal (ICCs), which are essentially the pacemaker cells of the gut. Amplitude, frequency, and energy delivered to the tissue are the important factors in determining tissue response.[4] Most investigators believe that stimulation occurs by having the electrodes excite the ICCs or the neural plexus.[5] An absence of these cells is thought to be seen in gastroparesis. One study found that 30% of patients with gastroparesis studied had depleted ICCs and those not depleted had a better response to therapy with GES.[6] A recent study found that patients with a higher proportion of ICCs had a better response to GES and symptomatic improvement than those with low numbers of ICCs.[7] Thus, to try and remedy the alterations in myoelectrical activity seen in gastroparesis, the device is placed in the patient's stomach and electrical current is delivered via electrodes to the gastric smooth muscle.

The use of neurostimulation of the gastrointestinal tract dates back to 1911 when William H. Dieffenbach placed electrodes rectally to try and treat constipation, ileus, and atony.[8] Then in 1963, Bilgutay and colleagues[9] attempted to treat postoperative ileus by placing electrodes via a nasogastric tube to help induce motility and cure patients of their ileus. In 1972, a study was done in canines that showed the ability to pace their gastrointestinal system using electrical stimulation.[10] That study was followed by the development of implantable pulse generators in the 1980s by Medtronic Inc. (Minneapolis, MN) for use in patients with abdominal pain and poor gastric motility.

Currently, there are 2 types of stimulation that have been hypothesized as ways to treat gastroparesis. One is a low-frequency, high-energy stimulation and the other is a high-frequency, low-energy stimulation.[4] The latter is the only option that is available commercially at this time. The frequency used is 12 cycles per minute, which is higher than the frequency of the intrinsic gastric slow wave of 3 cycles per minute. The device is marketed by Medtronic Inc. and is called the Enterra. Over time, studies have shown symptomatic benefits with use of GES in patients with gastroparesis. One study showed that patients with diabetic gastroparesis tended to have better response than those with idiopathic gastroparesis, men responded better than women, and those with more recent diagnoses of gastroparesis responded better than those with longer standing diagnoses[11] (**Fig. 1**).

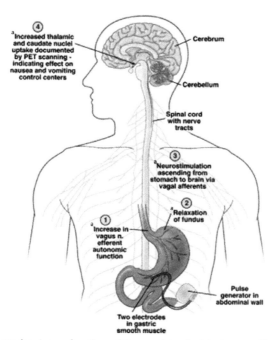

Fig. 1. Proposed mechanisms of action of the gastric electrical neurostimulator. [a] Demonstrated effects. (*From* Reddymasu SC, Sarosiek I, Mccallum RW. Severe gastroparesis: medical therapy or gastric electrical stimulation. Clin Gastroenterol Hepatol 2010;8(2):121; with permission.)

The GES can be implanted via laparotomy or laparoscopic surgery, the latter offering the advantage of a less invasive approach. The device consists of a pair of leads, a pulse generator, and a programming system.[4] The leads are placed in the muscularis propria of greater curvature of the stomach, about 10 cm proximal to the pylorus and connected to a pulse generator. The pulse generator is typically placed subcutaneously in the right or left upper quadrants of the abdomen. An external programming device controls the gastric stimulation parameters. The battery life is typically 5 to 10 years, but this duration can vary depending on the energy level settings. Patients often require higher energy settings, meaning the batteries will likely need to be changed at a shorter interval. Should the battery need to be changed, it can be done so without changing the electrodes. However, there has been a proposed development of a wireless GES, which would eliminate the need for battery changes[12] (**Figs. 2** and **3**).

To avoid the costs associated with GES as well as the risks associated with surgery or placement of a device that may ultimately not benefit the patient, some practitioners have implemented the use of temporary GES (tGES) to assess how a patient will respond to placement of a permanent GES. Although an off-label use for GES, there have been several studies that have shown symptomatic improvement with use of a tGES, which are discussed elsewhere in this article. This device can make the decision to proceed with invasive intervention easier for the patient. The electrodes can be placed endoscopically or via a percutaneous enteral gastrostomy tube (**Fig. 4**). Should the patient decide to proceed with permanent GES, a new pocket is made for pacemaker insertion and new leads are inserted in a different location of the stomach.[13]

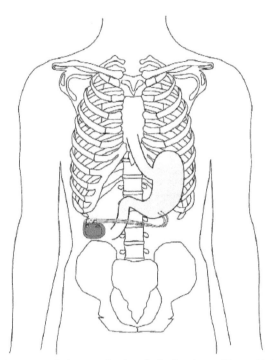

Fig. 2. Placement location of the gastric electrical stimulator. (*From* Abell T, Mccallum R, Hocking M, et al. Gastric electrical stimulation for medically refractory gastroparesis. Gastro-enterology 2003;125(2):422; with permission.)

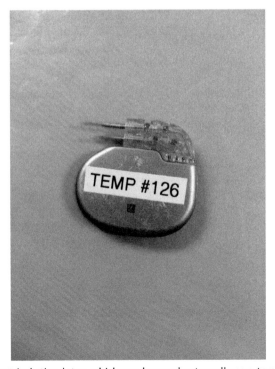

Fig. 3. Gastric electrical stimulator, which can be used externally as a temporary device.

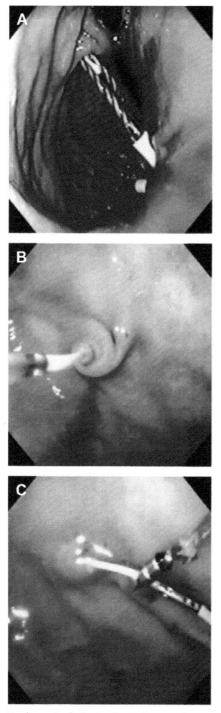

Fig. 4. (*A*) Endoscopic attachment of electrode to the gastric mucosa via a percutaneous enteral gastrostomy tract. (*B*) Temporary gastric stimulator electrode screwed into the gastric mucosa via endoscopy. (*C*) Anchoring of the electrode with the clip. (*From* Ayinala S, Batista O, Goyal A, et al. Temporary gastric electrical stimulation with orally or PEG-placed electrodes in patients with drug refractory gastroparesis. Gastrointest Endosc 2005;61(3):457; with permission.)

Further advancements in tGESs have even allowed for the placement of a device percutaneously (**Fig. 5**). The approach was developed in Sweden and could potentially allow for further minimally invasive therapies for patients with gastroparesis. One study showed promising results, with 22 of 27 patients having symptom reduction with placement of the device.[14]

Adverse Effects

Like any procedure and implanted device, a GES is not without possible adverse events, which can include[15]:

1. Dislodgment of the electrodes,
2. Lead migration or erosion,
3. Bowel obstruction,
4. Lead insulation damage,
5. Electrode penetration into the gastric mucosa, and
6. Infection.

Reasons that the GES would need to be removed include:

1. Infection,
2. Lack of improvement with GES,
3. Serious adverse effects as described (lead dislodgment, bowel obstruction, penetration into mucosa), and
4. Device migration.

Stimulator in Practice

The GEMS study, first published in 1997, was a short-term study in which 18 patients with permanent GES had an average 30 months of follow-up and showed improvement in nausea, vomiting, and quality of life.[16] The first double-blind study was published in 2003, with 33 patients with gastroparesis (17 diabetic and 16 idiopathic) who had high-frequency, low-amplitude GES placed. The study designers looked at patients after a 1-month "on" period, a 1-month "off" period, and then at 6 and 12 months. Their results were statistically significant for improvement in nausea and

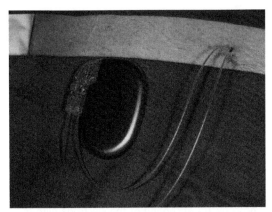

Fig. 5. Percutaneous placement of a gastric electrical stimulator. (*From* Abell TL, Chen J, Emmanuel A, et al. Neurostimulation of the gastrointestinal tract: review of recent developments. Neuromodulation 2015;18(3):223; with permission.)

vomiting when comparing the on versus off periods.[17] These results remained true at the 6- and 12-month follow-ups.

In a 2004 study, Lin and colleagues[18] examined 48 patients with refractory gastroparesis in which they performed long-term follow-up on patients with high-frequency GES. They found that patients' upper gastrointestinal symptoms improved, as well as glycemic control, health care-related quality of life, and nutritional status.[18]

In 2005, a study looked at the changes in the need for prokinetic/antiemetic medications, as well as the need for hospitalizations with patients with GES. This study looked at 37 gastroparetics (24 with diabetic gastroparesis, 8 with idiopathic gastroparesis, and 5 with postsurgical gastroparesis) who underwent GES implantation.[19] The study found a decrease in the use of daily antiemetic and/or prokinetic medications, with 27 patients on prokinetic medications before GES and 8 patients able to remain off of prokinetics at 1 year. Of the 26 patients on antiemetics before placement of GES, only 17 required antiemetics at 1 year. In addition to decreases in the need for medication, the study also demonstrated improvement in symptoms, quality of life, and frequency of hospitalizations. Looking at the year before implantation of GES, it was found that the average days spent in the hospital was 50 ± 10 days. After 1 year of GES, that figure improved significantly to 14 ± 3 days. These figures point to the improvements not only in symptoms and quality of life, but also to the decreased costs endured by patients with gastroparesis.

In a 2008 study, Brody and colleagues[20] studied 50 patients with gastroparesis and found that there was symptomatic improvement with gastric stimulation. The results of this study were significant for total symptom score improvement at 6 months ($P<.001$) and at 12 months ($P<.05$).[20] Again, we see promising results with GES for patients suffering from gastroparesis.

Many of these studies have focused on improvement in nausea and vomiting with GES. In 2013, a study was published that examined the use of GES to decrease abdominal pain in patients with gastroparesis. Ninety-five patients participated and 58 were reported to have severe pain, with the rest classified as nonsevere pain.[21] Of those with severe pain, their average pain scores decreased from 3.62 to 1.29 ($P<.001$) with tGES and with permanent GES their mean pain score was 2.30 ($P<.001$), still an improvement from their baseline.[21] For those with nonsevere pain, their average score decreased from 1.26 to 0.67 ($P = .01$) with tGES and went to 1.60 with permanent GES ($P = .221$).[21] Furthermore, there have been additional studies that have looked at the effects when the GES is set to 12 cycles per minute, which is about 4 times the intrinsic rate. Studies that have used this setting found not only long-term improvement, but also that patients' nausea and vomiting was improving within hours.[22]

Expanding the Scope of Gastric Electrical Stimulation

A cause of gastroparesis rarely seen is malignancy, known as malignancy-associated gastroparesis (MAG). Patients suffering from malignancy suffer from nausea and vomiting not amenable to typical antiemetics. Those who suffer from MAG experience significant morbidity from their condition. A study published in 2016 looked at patients with MAG receiving tGES. Although this study was limited in its sample size, it did find that patients with MAG experienced symptomatic improvement with tGES.[23]

There is a subset of patients who fall in to the category of gastroparesis-like syndrome. Patients with gastroparesis-like syndrome have the symptoms of those with gastroparesis (nausea, vomiting, abdominal pain, etc), but have normal gastric emptying studies. Given the improvement seen in patients with true gastroparesis, 1 study found that there was also improvement in those with gastroparesis-like syndrome with GES. Patients were separated into 3 groups based on their gastric emptying studies (delayed, normal, rapid) and they found that, after placement of a tGES, patients had a statistically significant (P<.001) improvement in nausea, vomiting, and overall total symptom scores.[24] More so, those with delayed emptying had more rapid emptying and those with rapid emptying slowed after placement of tGES.

In addition, GES can be used to treat other conditions. One study examined the use of GES in patients with cyclic vomiting syndrome. In this study, patients were found to have a 62% decrease in nausea from their baseline and an 83% decrease in vomiting with tGES, as well as a 46% decrease in nausea and 69% decrease in vomiting with permanent GES.[25] This finding demonstrates the versatility of the GES.

Temporary Gastric Electrical Stimulation

As discussed, some patients may opt to pursue placement of a tGES. The 2 routes that have been tested for placing electrodes are via a percutaneous enteral gastrostomy tube or endoscopically. A 2002 study examined 38 patients with drug-refractory gastroparesis. These patients underwent placement of a tGES and 33 of those who responded well ultimately had placement of a permanent GES. With the use of a GES, 97% of the patients reportedly experienced a greater than 80% decrease in nausea and vomiting, as well as an average weight gain of 5.5%. The results of this study were encouraging.[26]

In 2005, another study showed promising results for tGES. This study looked at the 2 methods for temporary stimulation and found that patients with refractory symptoms experienced a marked improvement with both modalities.[27] The 2 biggest factors in choosing to pursue tGES versus permanent GES was either the patient was too ill to undergo laparotomy or had issues with insurance reimbursement.

In 2011, a double-masked, randomized, placebo-controlled study taking place from 2005 to 2006 was published from the University of Mississippi and looked at continuous 72-hour temporary gastric electrical stimulation in 58 patients (38 idiopathic, 13 diabetes mellitus, 7 postoperative). These temporary stimulators were placed endoscopically. Patients were divided into 2 groups and one-half received stimulation in the first 4 days (group 1) and the other one-half received stimulation the second 4 days (group 2).[28] Symptom scores were assessed on a scale of 0 (none at all) to 4 (the most severe). As seen in **Table 1**, there was improvement in both nausea and vomiting with tGES. The advantage of tGES is that it can help clinicians to determine who might benefit and who might not benefit from the placement of a permanent stimulator. If patients do well with a temporary stimulator, then the next step would be to proceed with a permanent stimulator. However, if the patient does not improve, then they have now avoided an invasive surgery, as well as the costs associated with it by having the temporary stimulator placed instead of the invasive permanent stimulator.

After this study was completed, a long-term study followed it up to monitor how patients did with permanent gastric stimulation. The results of this study have yet to be published, until now. Of the 58 patients from the original study, 38 returned for permanent GES placement, with the rest excluded either owing to insurance issues or personal preference. There was about a 4-year average follow-up collected, with symptoms scores and gastric emptying studies obtained for each patient. The results are shown in **Fig. 6** and **Table 2**. There was improvement in symptoms scores and

Table 1
Symptom scores and gastric emptying results at baseline with follow-up at days 4 and 8 after placement of temporary gastric electrical stimulator

	Group 1 (On/Off)	Group 2 (Off/On)
Day 0 vomiting score[a]	1.82	2.68
Day 4 vomiting score[a]	0.29	1.37
Day 8 vomiting score	0.77	0.65
Day 0 nausea score	3.27	3.33
Day 4 nausea score	1.73	1.82
Day 8 nausea score	1.95	1.48
Day 0 total symptom score	12.77	14.57
Day 4 total symptom score	6.2	8.13
Day 8 total symptom score	7.00	6.26
Day 0 gastric emptying time, 1 h	67.07	66.13
Day 4 gastric emptying time, 1 h	69.96	62.35
Day 8 gastric emptying time, 1 h	64.71	68.67
Day 0 gastric emptying time, 2 h	46.74	37.41
Day 4 gastric emptying time, 2 h	46.85	38.00
Day 8 gastric emptying time, 2 h	42.19	40.92
Day 0 gastric emptying time, 4 h	24.70	16.43
Day 4 gastric emptying time, 4 h	24.11	21.85
Day 8 gastric emptying time, 4 h	24.71	20.25

Values are presented as the mean.
[a] Denotes a statically significant difference ($P<.05$) between the 2 groups.
Adapted from A double-masked, randomized, placebo-controlled trial of temporary endoscopic mucosal gastric electrical stimulation for gastroparesis. Gastrointest Endosc 2011;74:500; with permission.

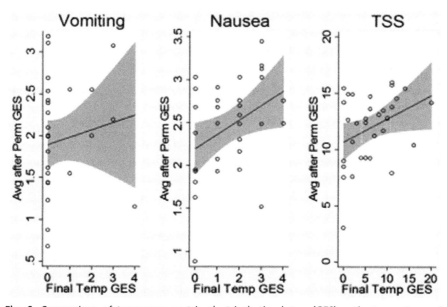

Fig. 6. Comparison of temporary gastric electrical stimulators (GES) patient symptoms at long-term follow-up. TSS, total symptoms score.

Table 2
Long-term follow-up of vomiting, nausea, total symptom scores, and gastric emptying times before stimulation and after both tGES and pGES

	Before GES		After tGES		Before pGES	
	Mean	Standard Deviation	Mean	Standard Deviation	Mean	Standard Deviation
Vomiting (0–4)	2.45	1.57	0.84	1.37	1.46	1.55
Nausea (0–4)	3.28	0.92	1.72	1.43	2.34	1.33
Total symptom scores (0–20)	14.00	3.51	7.2	5.66	11.21	5.90
GET 1 h %	67.89	22.15	69.39	21.40	63.94	22.61
GET 2 h %	43.92	26.34	44.89	28.39	40.35	28.20
GET 4 h %	22.03	27.17	27.64	29.95	20.41	26.89
GET total %	133.31	69.75	148.86	77.60	124.71	77.71

Abbreviations: GES, gastric electrical stimulator; GET, gastric emptying time; pGES, permanent gastric electrical stimulation; tGES, temporary gastric electrical stimulator.

gastric emptying times with placements of a permanent GES as compared with the patient's baseline. Seven patients were no longer delayed with permanent stimulation, whereas 10 patients were still delayed and 6 had newly delayed gastric emptying times after placement of the permanent GES. Those patients that were persistently or newly delayed may benefit from pyloric therapy.

Integrating Gastric Electrical Therapy and Pyloric Therapy

What if a patient does not improve with tGES? Or what if they fail to improve with permanent GES? There seems to be some thought that patients may have such severe gastric inflammation from their gastroparesis that they may not benefit from GES because the pylorus has become so stenosed that food is unable to pass. For these patients, the next step may be to open the pylorus via pyloroplasty, either surgically or gastric peroral endoscopic myotomy. One study showed that 40% of patients had loss of ICCs in the antrum, but that 70.5% of patients had depletion in ICCs in the pylorus.[29] This finding has allowed some of the focus to shift to the pylorus and advances have been made with gastric peroral endoscopic myotomy. In 2011, a study was published in which 26 patients underwent laparoscopic pyloroplasty with excellent outcomes, providing another treatment for those with refractory gastroparesis.[30] To minimize the invasiveness of the treatment of Gp, advancements have been made with the use of endoscopic means. In 2013, the first multicenter study in the United States using endoscopic myotomy was performed.[31] The patient was a 27-year-old woman with diabetic gastroparesis who was followed up at 12 weeks after the procedure. She had experienced improvement in her daily symptoms. **Fig. 7** details the stepwise process a clinician can use in treating gastroparesis. After a trial of tGES, the next step depends on the patient's response to therapy as to whether to proceed to permanent GES or pyloric therapy. Another option for those with refractory gastroparesis is a neuromuscular evaluation, which is a series of laboratory tests including paraneoplastic antibody panel, glutamic acid decarboxylase, thymidine phosphorylase, and free thymidine. It is thought that these patients may have antibodies that could be causing their symptoms and treatment can be immunomodulatory therapies with intravenous immunoglobulin.[32] Alternatively, there have been studies that have shown that some patients who have initial success with GES, but later redevelop symptoms

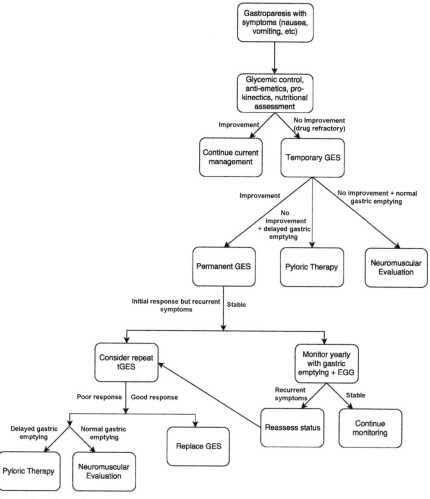

Fig. 7. Flowchart demonstrating stepwise treatment of patients with gastroparesis. EGG, electrogastrogram; GES, gastric electrical stimulator; tGES, temporary gastric electrical stimulator.

can benefit from surgical implantation of a new GES at different location.[13] Patients who are stable with placement of a GES can be monitored yearly with gastric emptying and electrogastrogram, which records the electrical signs of the stomach, similar to an electrocardiogram of the heart.

SUMMARY

Gastroparesis can be a severely debilitating disease and treatment is often difficult. Some patients experience frequent hospitalizations owing to the inability of treatment methods to control their nausea, vomiting, and pain. The development of the GES has revolutionized the way we treat gastroparesis. Patients have seen symptomatic improvement that has resulted in decreased hospitalizations. With the recent advancements seen in pyloric therapy, patients now have even more options for the treatment of their gastroparesis. A select subset of patients who are refractory may benefit from immunotherapy.

ACKNOWLEDGMENTS

The authors would like to thank the physicians and staff at the University of Mississippi Medical Center, including Dr Archana Kedar, Dr Michael Griswold, and Dr Christopher Lahr. The authors would like to thank the physicians and staff at the University of Louisville/Jewish Hospital GI Motility Clinic, including Dr Edmundo Rodriguez Frias who helped collect data for this article, as well as Dr Michael Hughes, Dr Abigail Stocker, Lindsay McElmurray PA-C, and Kelly Cooper NP. Last, the authors would like to thank Catherine McBride for her help with the article preparation.

REFERENCES

1. Williams PA, Nikitina Y, Kedar A, et al. Long-term effects of gastric stimulation on gastric electrical physiology. J Gastrointest Surg 2013;17:50–5 [discussion: p.55–6].
2. Bortolotti M. Gastric electrical stimulation for gastroparesis: a goal greatly pursued, but not yet attained. World J Gastroenterol 2011;17:273–82.
3. Huizinga JD, Lammers WJ. Gut peristalsis is governed by a multitude of cooperating mechanisms. Am J Physiol Gastrointest Liver Physiol 2009;296:G1–8.
4. Soffer EE. Gastric electrical stimulation for gastroparesis. J Neurogastroenterol Motil 2012;18:131–7.
5. Familoni BO, Abell TL, Gan Z, et al. Driving gastric electrical activity with electrical stimulation. Ann Biomed Eng 2005;33:356–64.
6. Forster J, Damjanov I, Lin Z, et al. Absence of the interstitial cells of Cajal in patients with gastroparesis and correlation with clinical findings. J Gastrointest Surg 2005;9:102–8.
7. Omer E, Kedar A, Nagarajarao H, et al. Cajal cell counts are important predictors of outcomes in drug refractory gastroparesis patients with neurostimulation. J Clin Gastroenterol 2018. [Epub ahead of print].
8. Dieffenbach WH. Electric treatment of intestinal obstruction and postoperative paralysis of the bowel. J Am Med Assoc 1911;LVI:958–9.
9. Bilgutay AM, Wingrove R, Griffen WO, et al. Gastro-intestinal pacing: a new concept in the treatment of ileus. Ann Surg 1963;158:338–48.
10. Kelly KA, La Force RC. Pacing the canine stomach with electric stimulation. Am J Physiol 1972;222:588–94.
11. Musunuru S, Beverstein G, Gould J. Preoperative predictors of significant symptomatic response after 1 year of gastric electrical stimulation for gastroparesis. World J Surg 2010;34:1853–8.
12. Deb S, Tang SJ, Abell TL, et al. An endoscopic wireless gastrostimulator (with video). Gastrointest Endosc 2012;75:411–5, 415.e1.
13. Harrison NS, Williams PA, Walker MR, et al. Evaluation and treatment of gastric stimulator failure in patients with gastroparesis. Surg Innov 2014;21:244–9.
14. Andersson S, Ringstrom G, Elfvin A, et al. Temporary percutaneous gastric electrical stimulation: a novel technique tested in patients with non-established indications for gastric electrical stimulation. Digestion 2011;83:3–12.
15. Parkman H. 1st edition. Gastroparesis: an issue of Gastroenterology Clinics of North America, vol. 44. Philadelphia: Elsevier Health Science; 2015.

16. Anand C, Al-Juburi A, Familoni B, et al. Gastric electrical stimulation is safe and effective: a long-term study in patients with drug-refractory gastroparesis in three regional centers. Digestion 2007;75:83–9.
17. Abell T, McCallum R, Hocking M, et al. Gastric electrical stimulation for medically refractory gastroparesis. Gastroenterology 2003;125:421–8.
18. Lin Z, Forster J, Sarosiek I, et al. Treatment of diabetic gastroparesis by high-frequency gastric electrical stimulation. Diabetes Care 2004;27:1071–6.
19. Lin Z, McElhinney C, Sarosiek I, et al. Chronic gastric electrical stimulation for gastroparesis reduces the use of prokinetic and/or antiemetic medications and the need for hospitalizations. Dig Dis Sci 2005;50:1328–34.
20. Brody F, Vaziri K, Saddler A, et al. Gastric electrical stimulation for gastroparesis. J Am Coll Surg 2008;207:533–8.
21. Lahr CJ, Griffith J, Subramony C, et al. Gastric electrical stimulation for abdominal pain in patients with symptoms of gastroparesis. Am Surg 2013;79:457–64.
22. Familoni BO, Abell TL, Bhaskar SK, et al. Gastric electrical stimulation has an immediate antiemetic effect in patients with gastroparesis. IEEE Trans Biomedical Eng 2006;53:1038–46.
23. Shah H, Wendorf G, Ahmed S, et al. Treating an oft-unrecognized and troublesome entity: using gastric electrical stimulation to reduce symptoms of malignancy-associated gastroparesis. Support Care Cancer 2017;25:27–31.
24. Singh S, McCrary J, Kedar A, et al. Temporary endoscopic stimulation in gastroparesis-like syndrome. J Neurogastroenterol Motil 2015;21:520–7.
25. Grover I, Kim R, Spree DC, et al. Gastric electrical stimulation is an option for patients with refractory cyclic vomiting syndrome. J Neurogastroenterol Motil 2016; 22:643–9.
26. Abell TL, Van Cutsem E, Abrahamsson H, et al. Gastric electrical stimulation in intractable symptomatic gastroparesis. Digestion 2002;66:204–12.
27. Ayinala S, Batista O, Goyal A, et al. Temporary gastric electrical stimulation with orally or PEG-placed electrodes in patients with drug refractory gastroparesis. Gastrointest Endosc 2005;61:455–61.
28. Abell TL, Johnson WD, Kedar A, et al. A double-masked, randomized, placebo-controlled trial of temporary endoscopic mucosal gastric electrical stimulation for gastroparesis. Gastrointest Endosc 2011;74:496–503.e3.
29. Moraveji S, Bashashati M, Elhanafi S, et al. Depleted interstitial cells of Cajal and fibrosis in the pylorus: novel features of gastroparesis. Neurogastroenterol Motil 2016;28:1048–54.
30. Hibbard ML, Dunst CM, Swanstrom LL. Laparoscopic and endoscopic pyloroplasty for gastroparesis results in sustained symptom improvement. J Gastrointest Surg 2011;15:1513–9.
31. Khashab MA, Ngamruengphong S, Carr-Locke D, et al. Gastric per-oral endoscopic myotomy for refractory gastroparesis: results from the first multicenter study on endoscopic pyloromyotomy (with video). Gastrointest Endosc 2017; 85:123–8.
32. Ashat M, Lewis A, Liaquat H, et al. Intravenous immunoglobulin in drug and device refractory patients with the symptoms of gastroparesis-an open-label study. Neurogastroenterol Motil 2018;30(3). https://doi.org/10.1111/nmo.13256.

Surgical Management for Gastroparesis

Ahmed M. Zihni, MD, MPH[a], Christy M. Dunst, MD[a],
Lee L. Swanström, MD, FRCSEng[a,b,*]

KEYWORDS

- Laparoscopy • Gastroparesis • Endoscopy • Pyloromyotomy • Per oral myotomy
- POP • Pyloroplasty • Gastric stimulation

KEY POINTS

- Gastroparesis is increasing in incidence and is multifactorial.
- A significant proportion of patients fail conservative treatment and will need interventions.
- A stepwise approach to surgical therapy is needed: POP, pyloroplasty, gastric nerve stimulator, subtotal gastrectomy.
- Multimodal approaches may have a place.

INTRODUCTION

Gastroparesis syndrome is defined by nausea, vomiting, bloating, or abdominal pain in the context of objectively delayed gastric emptying (DGE) without mechanical gastric outlet obstruction. Currently, there is no definitive cure for gastroparesis, and the goals of management are strictly palliative, although correction of underlying pathologic conditions may decrease symptoms. Gastroparesis is most commonly idiopathic, but well-described diabetes-related and postoperative variants are prevalent as well.[1] Its pathophysiology, as it is currently understood, involves the derangement of the complex interplay of factors regulating normal gastric motility, including injury or degenerative changes to the vagus nerves, uncoupling of electric signaling and mechanical effects in the gastric muscles, derangement of gastrointestinal (GI) hormones, depletion of the interstitial cells of Cajal, and the chronic effects of prolonged food bezoar presence in the stomach.[2,3] The current prevalence of gastroparesis is estimated at 4% of the population, and it is widely perceived to be an

The authors report no disclosures relevant to this topic and received no compensation for writing this.
[a] Division of GI/MIS, The Oregon Clinic, 4805 Northeast Glisan, 6N60, Portland, OR 97213, USA;
[b] IHU-Strasbourg, 1 Place de l'Hôpital, 67000 Strasbourg, France
* Corresponding author. Division of GI/MIS, The Oregon Clinic, Oregon Health and Science University, 4805 Northeast Glisan, 6N60, Portland, OR 97213.
E-mail address: lswanstrom@gmail.com

Gastrointest Endoscopy Clin N Am 29 (2019) 85–95
https://doi.org/10.1016/j.giec.2018.08.006
1052-5157/19/© 2018 Elsevier Inc. All rights reserved.

increasing diagnosis.[1] Many patients with gastroparesis have only mild symptoms that can usually be managed by dietary modification, antiemetics, antacids, and motility agents. In some patients, the condition is transient, resolving after weeks, months, or years, but in the majority it is more or less permanent. A significant subset of patients, with severe or progressive disease, can go on to require operative intervention to reduce symptoms and improve quality of life. In this article, the authors review a surgical treatment algorithm for gastroparesis as well as the techniques and current evidence surrounding common and emerging surgical modalities for this disease.

SURGICAL ALGORITHM

Management algorithms for the medical and surgical treatment of gastroparesis have yet to be established with sufficient evidence and consensus to be definitive. Here, the authors present their group's treatment algorithm, derived from extensive experience (**Fig. 1**).

First, the authors verify that the patient meets clinical and diagnostic criteria for gastroparesis, including ruling out mechanical gastric outflow obstruction or reversible exogenous causes, and confirm that symptom severity and patient expectations are appropriate to proceed with surgery. Interestingly, only 10% of patients referred for surgical consideration of gastroparesis have severe nutritional impairment. These patients are offered enteral jejunal feeding access to optimize nutrition before any

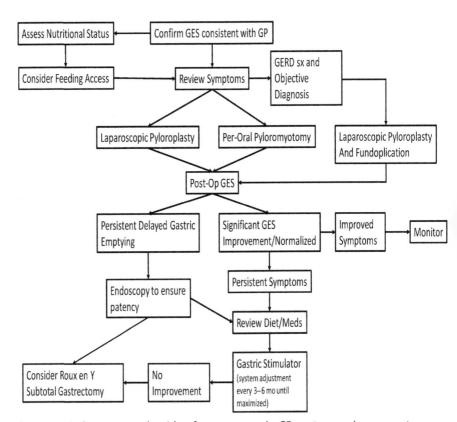

Fig. 1. Surgical treatment algorithm for gastroparesis. GP, gastroparesis; sx, symptom.

surgical treatment is attempted. Rarely, central venous access is also established to assist patients in achieving adequate hydration or for total parenteral nutrition in cases where there is generalized gut dysmotility.

Mandatory diagnostic workup includes an upper GI barium study to define anatomy and rule out mechanical obstruction, an upper endoscopy with biopsies to rule out infiltrative gastric malignancy, *Helicobacter pylori*, gastroesophageal reflux disease (GERD), or other associated pathologic condition, and assessing solid food retention and a quantitative gastric-emptying study (GES), either a 4-hour radionuclide examination or a gastric-emptying capsule study. The latter is both to confirm the diagnosis and to serve as a baseline measurement for future follow-up. The patient should have a comprehensive medical evaluation, and all potential underlying pathologic conditions (diabetes, narcotic addiction, pathologic eating behaviors, and so forth) should be corrected as much as possible.

The authors' first-line surgical therapy has traditionally been laparoscopic pyloroplasty, although their group and others are increasingly using per oral pyloromyotomy (POP) to improve gastric outflow at the pylorus. Fundoplication at the time of pyloroplasty is often an important adjunct in patients with coexistent objective GERD. Three months after pyloroplasty or POP, a repeat GES is performed to objectively assess improvement. Patients with improved symptoms and gastric emptying continue long-term medical management and monitoring. Patients with persistent delayed emptying were evaluated endoscopically to rule out gastric outlet obstruction as a result of inadequate pyloroplasty or extensive scar or stricture. If this is ruled out, they are usually offered gastric neurostimulation for persistent nausea. The final step of the algorithm for patients with symptoms refractory to all of the above treatments is laparoscopic near-total gastrectomy. Symptoms may persist even after gastrectomy, due to global GI motility anomalies that can accompany gastroparesis. There are no surgical treatments available to these patients beyond providing enteral feeding access to those who need it. Concurrent gastric stimulation and pyloroplasty or upfront gastrectomy is used is select cases.

LAPAROSCOPIC PYLOROPLASTY

Pyloroplasty has long been the mainstay surgical approach to improve gastric emptying. The pyloroplasty is designed to improve gastric emptying by dividing the pyloric muscle, which can serve as an obstruction, and by increasing the cross-sectional area of the gastric outlet.

The multiple invasive options available should be discussed with the patient (see **Fig. 1**). In most cases, the authors would recommend a laparoscopic pyloroplasty as the first line of treatment. Laparoscopic pyloroplasty is performed according to the principles of the Heineke-Mikulicz pyloroplasty. Laparoscopic access is established with ports positioned to triangulate the pylorus and retract the liver. A partial Kocher maneuver is performed to mobilize and expose the pylorus and proximal duodenum. The pylorus is identified by palpation or by endoscopic transillumination if needed, and a 5-cm gastroduodenostomy is created across the pylorus longitudinally using scissors or ultrasonic shears (**Fig. 2**). The resulting defect is then closed transversely using running absorbable sutures. A second row of sutures may be used to imbricate this suture line. Afterward, endoscopy is performed to ensure patency and test the suture line integrity using gas or methylene blue.

Postoperatively, the authors' practice is for patients to undergo contrast upper GI radiography on postoperative day 1 to confirm adequate emptying through the pyloroplasty. Subsequently, their diet is advanced to clear and then full liquids, which are

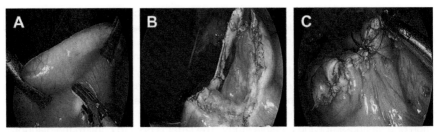

Fig. 2. Laparoscopic pyloroplasty. (*A*) The pylorus is identified. (*B*) Full-thickness longitudinal enterotomy is created. (*C*) Enterotomy is closed transversely.

continued for 2 weeks. The authors routinely prescribe a proton pump inhibitor for 6 to 8 weeks postoperatively to allow the incision to heal. A GES is performed at 3 months to evaluate the impact of the surgery on gastric emptying.

Complications specifically associated with laparoscopic pyloroplasty are rare but include gastric outlet obstruction caused by inadvertently including the back wall of the pylorus in the suture line (early) or stricture (late). "Backwalling" is generally not full thickness and can be opened relatively easily endoscopically. If not, it can be managed expectantly with decompressive gastrostomy tube and feeding jejunostomy for a few months until the suture absorbs. Leakage from the suture line, which could manifest as abdominal sepsis or contained abscess, is the most serious complication. Depending on the timing and severity of the leak, reoperation or percutaneous drainage may be indicated for source control along with antibiotics. Another associated complication is pyloric stricture with obstruction, which is very rare and best treated with near-total gastrectomy rather than revision.

The outcomes of pyloroplasty in patients with gastroparesis have been relatively well studied. Pyloric compliance and diameter as measured by impedance planimetry have been shown experimentally to be linked to gastroparesis symptoms, confirming the proposed mechanism of the pyloroplasty's therapeutic effect.[4] The authors' group performed a large retrospective review of 6-month outcomes in patients who underwent laparoscopic pyloroplasty and noted statistically significant improvements in Gastroparesis Cardinal Symptom Index (GCSI) scores, and objective improvement of gastric emptying in 86% of patients with normalization occurring in 77% of patients.[5] The broader literature supports these findings, with several short- and medium-term reports from various groups reporting some degree of symptom improvement in 80% to 95% of patients, improvement of gastric emptying in 80% to 96% of patients, and normalization of gastric emptying in 60% to 77% of patients.[6–9] Long-term data for the efficacy of pyloroplasty are less robust, although the authors' group has shown that at 10 years symptomatic improvement is sustained in up to 80% of patients, although in their cohort more than a third of patients eventually required an adjunct procedure along with their pyloroplasty.[10]

PER ORAL PYLOROMYOTOMY

POP is a technique for dividing the pyloric muscle endoscopically (**Fig. 3**). POP emerged from the techniques of submucosal dissection pioneered for use in submucosal esophageal and gastric tumor excision and per oral endoscopic myotomy. It has the advantages of shorter length of hospital stay and less postoperative pain compared with laparoscopic pyloroplasty.[11]

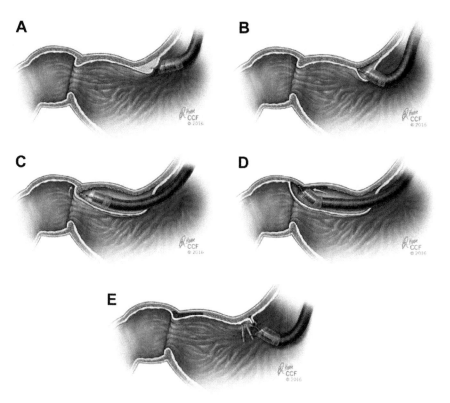

Fig. 3. POP. (*A*) Submucosal injection. (*B*, *C*) Creation of submucosal tunnel. (*D*) Pyloromyotomy. (*E*) Clip closure of mucosotomy. (*Courtesy of* Cleveland Clinic Foundation, Cleveland, OH; with permission.)

POP is usually performed in an operating room in case conversion to laparoscopic or open surgery is necessary. It is always performed under general anesthesia with endotracheal intubation. A diagnostic endoscopy is first performed to identify anatomic landmarks and clear the stomach of retained food. A dissecting cap is affixed to the gastroscope tip, which is used to deflect away the mucosa and create tension during submucosal dissection. A point 3 to 5 cm proximal to the pylorus is identified, and 5 to 10 mL of lifting solution is injected into the submucosa at this position to separate the mucosa from the submucosal and serosal structures below. A mucosotomy is created in the lifted mucosa, just large enough to allow the gastroscope to enter, and a submucosal tunnel is created by dividing submucosal areolar tissue using electrocautery. The dissection has been described along either the lesser or the greater curves. It is carried to the pylorus, which is visualized endoscopically as a thick white band of muscle. The dissection is carried just beyond the pylorus until duodenal mucosa is encountered. The pylorus is next divided using electrocautery, and the scope is retracted with closure of the mucosotomy using endoscopic clips or endoscopic suturing.[11]

Postoperatively, contrast upper GI radiography may be used to rule out full-thickness perforation. Patients are then advanced to a full liquid diet, which is maintained for 2 weeks, and discharged home. Patients are generally admitted overnight, although discharged on the day of surgery after POP has been described. Patients are discharged on proton pump inhibitors for 6 to 8 weeks and undergo GES at 3 months as described after laparoscopic pyloroplasty. Complications after POP are rare but include endoluminal GI bleeding, full-thickness perforation, and inadequate myotomy requiring reoperation.

POP has not been studied as extensively as laparoscopic pyloroplasty, but emerging data reveal promising trends. The authors' group published an early series of the procedure in which symptomatic improvement was observed in 86% of patients, and improvement of gastric emptying was noted at 3 months as well.[12] In a larger series of POP, 4-hour gastric emptying was found to improve significantly from 63% to 80% at 3 months, as well as a significant improvement from 4.6 to 3.3 in the GCSI over the same period.[13] These early data and ongoing studies into the use of POP suggest that this procedure will play an important role in the treatment of gastroparesis in the future.

GASTRIC NEUROSTIMULATOR

The gastric neurostimulator is an implantable device that delivers an intermittent high-frequency electrical impulse to the smooth muscle of the stomach. The precise mechanism of the gastric stimulation is not fully understood but is thought to involve direct action of the electric impulse on the muscle as well as interaction with vagal fibers.[14] Stimulators are generally implanted in a combined laparoscopic (lead implantation) and open (generator placement) technique and can also be performed with robotic assistance if the surgeon has trouble with suturing the leads. First, the 2 stimulator leads are introduced into the abdomen laparoscopically. They are implanted on the greater curve 10 to 12 cm proximal to the pylorus, a few millimeters from the edge of the greater curvature, by tunneling them 2.5 cm through the subserosa of the gastric wall (**Fig. 4**). The leads are placed 1 cm apart in a parallel configuration and then secured in place using fasteners and permanent sutures. Endoscopy is performed to confirm that the leads are not intraluminal. The leads are brought out of the abdomen through one of the laparoscopic ports. A subcutaneous pocket is then created at the site where the leads emerge from the abdomen and the stimulator and battery construct is placed in this pocket and secured to the fascia with permanent sutures. Using an interrogator, the stimulator is activated and programmed to nominal values of impedance, current, and voltage. Skin incisions are closed, and the operation is concluded.

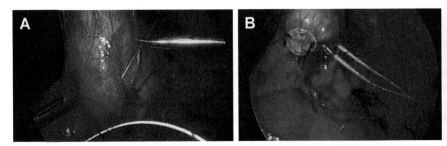

Fig. 4. Laparoscopic neurostimulator insertion. (A) The greater curve is identified 12 cm proximal to the pylorus, and needles are used to create a tunnel for the stimulator leads 1 cm apart. (B) The stimulator leads are implanted into the gastric wall and fastened in place using sutures and reinforcing discs. Of note, this patient has a venting gastrostomy tube in place along the greater curve; its bumper is noted in image (B).

Postoperatively, patients are rapidly advanced to a regular diet and discharged home. The authors generally perform stimulator implantation as an outpatient procedure. At 3 months, the stimulator is interrogated, and the current may be increased as needed every 3 months until symptoms are substantially improved or the maximal current is reached. Commercially available neurostimulators have a battery of life of 5 to 8 years and have to be replaced when they stop functioning. Replacement is done in the operating room by reopening the skin at the site of stimulator implantation, removing the stimulator, and replacing it with a new one that is reconnected to the leads already in place. In most cases, there is no need to reenter the abdomen unless the leads are disrupted. Complications of laparoscopic gastric stimulator placement include cardiopulmonary complications of general anesthesia, inadvertent injury to surrounding structures, bowel obstruction associated with the leads, lead perforation, pain or migration at the implantation site, or infection of the device necessitating replacement.

Although the mechanism of action of neurostimulation on the gastroparetic stomach has not yet been fully worked out, the efficacy of the treatment has been examined in several studies. In an elegant randomized controlled trial, a large cohort of subjects all received a neurostimulator but had it intermittently activated or deactivated during separate phases of the study in a blinded manner. It was found that during periods when the stimulator was on, patients experienced significant reductions in vomiting and overall symptom scores of up to 80% as well as some improvement in objectively measured gastric emptying.[14] These effects have been confirmed in several other prospective and retrospective reports.[15–18]

LAPAROSCOPIC GASTRECTOMY

Gastrectomy in some regards seems an illogical treatment for the gastroparetic. On the other hand, it is often the only thing to offer patients who have failed all other medical and surgical treatments as described above or even sometimes as first-line therapy. Gastrectomy, total or subtotal, is the most definitive and radical surgical modality available and represents the "end of the road" for surgical treatment of gastroparesis. In the authors' practice, they generally offer patients a laparoscopic near-total gastrectomy with Roux-en-Y reconstruction (**Fig. 5**). This procedure can also be performed via open or robot-assisted approaches, although laparoscopic is the gold standard. The stomach is mobilized, and all of its vascular pedicles are divided except for the left gastric artery, which is preserved. The duodenum is divided just distal to the pylorus. A small gastric pouch is created by stapling and dividing the stomach from the lesser curve just distal to the left gastric artery insertion toward the angle of His. Next, a length of small bowel distal to the ligament of Treitz is selected that allows for easy reach to the gastric pouch in the antecolic position. The small bowel is divided at this point and the Roux limb is brought into the upper abdomen and anastomosed to the gastric pouch using a circular stapler. A jejunojejunostomy is then created using

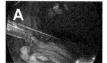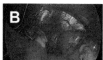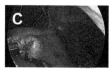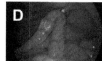

Fig. 5. Laparoscopic subtotal gastrectomy. (*A*) Division of the stomach distal to the left gastric artery. (*B*) Gastrojejunostomy. (*C*) Creation of jejunojejunostomy using linear stapler. (*D*) Adjunctive J-tube is often necessary.

a linear stapler to create a typical 60- to 75-cm Roux limb. The specimen is removed. All mesenteric defects are then closed using permanent suture, and endoscopy is performed to confirm patent anastomosis and perform leak testing.

Patients are evaluated with contrast upper GI radiography on the first postoperative day, and drain amylase is checked (if a drain is placed). If no leak is noted, patients are advanced to clear liquids and then a pureed diet, which they continue for 2 weeks. Drains are removed before discharge. Near-total gastrectomy is a more radical surgical approach than others described in this article and does bear a higher risk profile. The authors' group and others have reported an anastomotic leak rate of nearly 10% and reoperation rate of 17% for this complicated patient group.[19] Other complications include bleeding, infection, bowel obstructions due to adhesive disease or internal hernia at the mesenteric defects, and refractory symptoms due to global dysmotility or Roux limb syndrome. Occasionally, even the tiny gastric remnant becomes the focus of persistent gastroparesis symptoms necessitating completion gastrectomy and esophagojejunostomy. Despite the complication profile, laparoscopic subtotal gastrectomy has been well studied and shown to be efficacious in patients with gastroparesis. The authors' group reported symptomatic improvement in up to 89% of patients after gastrectomy for refractory gastroparesis, and reports from other groups seem to indicate symptomatic benefit as well.[15,19–24]

ENTERAL ACCESS

Enteral feeding and venting tubes can play a role in the management of gastroparesis. Both gastrostomy and jejunostomy tubes are used in this patient population. Gastrostomy is used for venting the stomach, often in patients with gastroparesis refractory to other medical and surgical therapy who are not yet ready for gastrectomy. These tubes can be placed laparoscopically but are most commonly inserted percutaneously with endoscopic guidance. The use of percutaneous endoscopic gastrostomy (PEG) for venting has been studied as a palliative measure for a variety of processes, including malignant bowel obstruction and gastroparesis, and has been shown to be efficacious in relieving symptoms such as nausea and bloating, although most series to date have been small.[25–28] The authors do not typically use decompressive gastrostomy tubes as definitive treatment of gastroparesis. In their practice, this is usually an adjunctive measure to help patients in the early postoperative healing phase or for those who ultimately undergo gastrectomy. Nearly all patients who have a decompressive PEG are liberated from it after they recover from pyloroplasty and/or gastric stimulator implantation.

Jejunal access is used for feeding in patients with gastroparesis who require nutritional support. Jejunal access can be achieved through a nasojejunal tube or a transcutaneous jejunal tube (J-tube). In the authors' practice, they generally perform laparoscopic J-tube placement, which can be done as a stand-alone procedure in severely malnourished patients to allow them to undergo nutritional optimization before further surgical interventions, or at the same time as a pyloroplasty or subtotal gastrectomy. The authors generally avoid placing feeding tubes during a laparoscopic neurostimulator insertion due to the theoretic risk of implant infection. Laparoscopic jejunostomy placement involves identifying a loop of jejunum that reaches the abdominal wall without tension, then affixing it with transfascial stitches to the abdominal wall, and then creating a jejunostomy using a wire-guided dilator with peel-away sheath. The J-tube must remain in place for at least 1 month to allow an epithelialized tract to form. A full discussion of long-term J-tube management and feeding strategies is beyond the scope of this article, but liberation from tube feeding and transition to oral diet are the long-term goals for all patients with gastroparesis. The authors have found that only 8% of gastroparesis patients referred to their practice require enteral feeding access, and that 55% of them are ultimately able to be liberated from tube feeding. Pyloroplasty is associated with successful liberation from tube feeding.[29]

LAPAROSCOPIC FUNDOPLICATION

Fundoplication is an important part of the gastroparesis treatment algorithm. It is known that fundoplication alone can improve gastric emptying, and it is an important adjunctive procedure in patients with both GERD and gastroparesis.[30] GERD in gastroparesis patients can be due to gastric overflow from a dilated poorly emptying stomach or may be a separate process unrelated to the patient's motility. Because the symptom complexes of the 2 disorders overlap, a high index of suspicion must be maintained for the presence of both disorders. In patients referred for GERD who exhibit significant symptoms of nausea, vomiting, or bloating, a GES should be performed along with the standard prefundoplication workup. A significant retained food bezoar identified during preoperative endoscopy in preparation for endoscopy is also suggestive for gastroparesis. Patients referred for gastroparesis who complain of significant heartburn, regurgitation, or dysphagia should undergo comprehensive objective GERD evaluation, including esophagogastroduodenoscopy, pH, and manometry studies. Although a full fundoplication is not contraindicated, consideration is taken for a partial fundoplication and/or concurrent temporary venting gastrostomy tube in this difficult population due to the risk of early wrap herniation. The authors have found this to be an effective strategy in high-risk patients.

When both GERD and gastroparesis are identified, a laparoscopic fundoplication along with pyloroplasty are performed as the first-line treatment. The technical details of the fundoplication vary depending on which wrap is performed, but in most cases, a full hiatal dissection is performed; any hiatal hernias are repaired with permanent sutures and bolstered with an absorbable synthetic mesh if necessary. The greater curve is mobilized enough to allow an antireflux wrap to be constructed without undue tension. Once this is accomplished, pyloroplasty is performed as described above.

Laparoscopic fundoplication and pyloroplasty have been well studied, and results are generally very favorable for this procedure in patients with coexistent GERD and gastroparesis. Farrell and colleagues[30] demonstrated that a full fundoplication led to a 38% improvement in gastric emptying at 1 year, but adding a pyloroplasty increased the level of improvement to 70%. Masqusi and Velanovich[8] showed that patients who underwent fundoplication and pyloroplasty experienced excellent levels of reflux control similar to extensive published literature on antireflux surgery as well as an 80% reduction in bloating symptoms in those with abnormal gastric emptying preoperatively. The authors' group performed a large retrospective study of patients with and without symptoms and objective evidence of DGE who underwent antireflux fundoplication and discovered that although GERD symptoms reliably improved after fundoplication regardless of DGE status, these symptoms persisted in patients who underwent fundoplication alone but were significantly improved in those who also had a pyloroplasty.[31]

SUMMARY

Gastroparesis remains a challenging disorder, one who's pathophysiology is still not fully understood. Medical treatment algorithms continue to evolve. The role of surgery is also evolving, as new procedures emerge and more robust outcomes data sharpen the understanding of their use. In this review, the authors presented their current surgical treatment algorithm for this disease, an overview of commonly performed operations, and current data regarding their outcomes.

REFERENCES

1. Jung HK. The incidence, prevalence, and survival of gastroparesis in olmsted county, Minnesota, 1996-2006 (gastroenterology 2009;136:1225-1233). J Neurogastroenterol Motil 2010;16:99–100.
2. Reddymasu SC, Sarosiek I, McCallum RW. Severe gastroparesis: medical therapy or gastric electrical stimulation. Clin Gastroenterol Hepatol 2010;8:117–24.
3. Grover M, Bernard CE, Pasricha PJ, et al. Clinical-histological associations in gastroparesis: results from the Gastroparesis Clinical Research Consortium. Neurogastroenterol Motil 2012;24:531–9, e249.
4. Gourcerol G, Tissier F, Melchior C, et al. Impaired fasting pyloric compliance in gastroparesis and the therapeutic response to pyloric dilatation. Aliment Pharmacol Ther 2015;41:360–7.
5. Shada AL, Dunst CM, Pescarus R, et al. Laparoscopic pyloroplasty is a safe and effective first-line surgical therapy for refractory gastroparesis. Surg Endosc 2016;30:1326–32.
6. Hibbard ML, Dunst CM, Swanstrom LL. Laparoscopic and endoscopic pyloroplasty for gastroparesis results in sustained symptom improvement. J Gastrointest Surg 2011;15:1513–9.
7. Mancini SA, Angelo JL, Peckler Z, et al. Pyloroplasty for refractory gastroparesis. Am Surg 2015;81:738–46.
8. Masqusi S, Velanovich V. Pyloroplasty with fundoplication in the treatment of combined gastroesophageal reflux disease and bloating. World J Surg 2007;31: 332–6.
9. Toro JP, Lytle NW, Patel AD, et al. Efficacy of laparoscopic pyloroplasty for the treatment of gastroparesis. J Am Coll Surg 2014;218:652–60.
10. Abdelmoaty WF, Dunst CM, Zihni AM, et al. Ten Year Outcomes of Pyloroplasty in Adult Gastroparesis. Surg Endosc 2018. [Epub ahead of print].
11. Allemang MT, Strong AT, Haskins IN, et al. How I do it: per-oral pyloromyotomy (POP). J Gastrointest Surg 2017;21:1963–8.
12. Shlomovitz E, Pescarus R, Cassera MA, et al. Early human experience with per-oral endoscopic pyloromyotomy (POP). Surg Endosc 2015;29:543–51.
13. Rodriguez JH, Haskins IN, Strong AT, et al. Per oral endoscopic pyloromyotomy for refractory gastroparesis: initial results from a single institution. Surg Endosc 2017;31:5381–8.
14. Abell T, McCallum R, Hocking M, et al. Gastric electrical stimulation for medically refractory gastroparesis. Gastroenterology 2003;125:421–8.
15. Arthur LE, Slattery L, Richardson W. Tailored approach to gastroparesis significantly improves symptoms. Surg Endosc 2018;32:977–82.
16. de Csepel J, Goldfarb B, Shapsis A, et al. Electrical stimulation for gastroparesis. Gastric motility restored. Surg Endosc 2006;20:302–6.
17. McCallum RW, Sarosiek I, Parkman HP, et al. Gastric electrical stimulation with Enterra therapy improves symptoms of idiopathic gastroparesis. Neurogastroenterol Motil 2013;25:815–24.
18. Timratana P, El-Hayek K, Shimizu H, et al. Laparoscopic gastric electrical stimulation for medically refractory diabetic and idiopathic gastroparesis. J Gastrointest Surg 2013;17:461–70.

19. Bhayani NH, Sharata AM, Dunst CM, et al. End of the road for a dysfunctional end organ: laparoscopic gastrectomy for refractory gastroparesis. J Gastrointest Surg 2015;19:411–7.
20. Borrazzo EC. Surgical management of gastroparesis: gastrostomy/jejunostomy tubes, gastrectomy, pyloroplasty, gastric electrical stimulation. J Gastrointest Surg 2013;17:1559–61.
21. Jones MP, Maganti K. A systematic review of surgical therapy for gastroparesis. Am J Gastroenterol 2003;98:2122–9.
22. Rivera RE, Eagon JC, Soper NJ, et al. Experience with laparoscopic gastric resection: results and outcomes for 37 cases. Surg Endosc 2005;19:1622–6.
23. Sarosiek I, Davis B, Eichler E, et al. Surgical approaches to treatment of gastroparesis: gastric electrical stimulation, pyloroplasty, total gastrectomy and enteral feeding tubes. Gastroenterol Clin North Am 2015;44:151–67.
24. Sun Z, Rodriguez J, McMichael J, et al. Surgical treatment of medically refractory gastroparesis in the morbidly obese. Surg Endosc 2015;29:2683–9.
25. DeEulis TG, Yennurajalingam S. Venting gastrostomy at home for symptomatic management of bowel obstruction in advanced/recurrent ovarian malignancy: a case series. J Palliat Med 2015;18:722–8.
26. Mohammed AM, Dennis RJ. Use of a venting PEG tube in the management of recurrent acute gastric dilatation associated with Prader-Willi syndrome. J Surg Case Rep 2016;1:1–2.
27. Shaw C, Bassett RL, Fox PS, et al. Palliative venting gastrostomy in patients with malignant bowel obstruction and ascites. Ann Surg Oncol 2013;20:497–505.
28. Teriaky A, Gregor J, Chande N. Percutaneous endoscopic gastrostomy tube placement for end-stage palliation of malignant gastrointestinal obstructions. Saudi J Gastroenterol 2012;18:95–8.
29. Filicori F, Dunst CM, Zihni AM, et al. Patient characteristics associated with successful cessation of tube feeds in malnourished patients with gastroparesis. Gastrointest Surg 2018. [Epub ahead of print].
30. Farrell TM, Richardson WS, Halkar R, et al. Nissen fundoplication improves gastric motility in patients with delayed gastric emptying. Surg Endosc 2001; 15:271–4.
31. Khajanchee YS, Dunst CM, Swanstrom LL. Outcomes of Nissen fundoplication in patients with gastroesophageal reflux disease and delayed gastric emptying. Arch Surg 2009;144:823–8.

Botulinum Toxin Injection for Treatment of Gastroparesis

Trisha S. Pasricha, MD[a], Pankaj J. Pasricha, MD[b],*

KEYWORDS

- Botulinum neurotoxin • BOTOX • Gastroparesis • Pyloric dysfunction
- Pylorospasm

KEY POINTS

- Botulinum toxin injections for gastroparesis are based on the hypothesis that amelioration of pyloric dysfunction among a subset of patients will lead to symptomatic improvement.
- Although several open-label studies showed initial promise, no data exist demonstrating causality between pyloric dysfunction and symptoms of gastroparesis.
- Two randomized clinical trials have failed to demonstrate a difference in clinical outcomes between botulinum toxin versus placebo in gastroparesis.
- Based on current evidence, further use of botulinum toxin for gastroparesis is discouraged outside of a research setting.

INTRODUCTION

Refractory gastroparesis is a challenging disorder characterized by symptoms of nausea, vomiting, early satiety, post-prandial fullness, and abdominal pain for which viable effective treatment options are scarce.[1,2] Although the cause of most cases remains idiopathic, gastroparesis has known associations with diabetes mellitus and with prior surgery. Clinicians will likely continue to see an increase in gastroparesis as the incidence of the metabolic syndrome increases worldwide. One relatively safe intervention, injection of botulinum neurotoxin (BoNT) in the pylorus, has been controversial but still widely practiced. In this article, the authors review pyloric dysfunction in gastroparesis, BoNT as a therapeutic modality, and its potential use in gastroparesis based on the latest literature.

Disclosure Statement: The authors have no relevant commercial or financial conflicts of interest. This work was partially supported by a grant from the NIH to P.J. Pasricha (DK073983).
[a] Osler Medical Training Program, Department of Medicine, Johns Hopkins Hospital, 1800 Orleans Street, Baltimore, MD 21287, USA; [b] Department of Gastroenterology, Johns Hopkins Hospital, Ross 958, 720 Rutland Avenue, Baltimore, MD 21205, USA
* Corresponding author.
E-mail address: ppasric1@jhmi.edu

PYLORIC DYSFUNCTION IN GASTROPARESIS

When Mearin and colleagues[3] first described pyloric dysfunction in diabetic gastroparesis in 1986, the pathogenesis and pathophysiology of the disease were poorly understood (it arguably remains so today). Historical studies had demonstrated a link between delayed gastric emptying and diabetes and early therapeutic approaches consisted of "prokinetic" agents, such as with domperidone or metoclopramide.[4–8] These drugs seemed initially promising, but rarely provided long-term "curative" solutions for patients suffering from clinical gastroparesis. Given a pathognomonic lack of mechanical obstruction in these patients, it was hypothesized that pyloric dysfunction may be a component of their overall upper gut dysmotility, contributing to symptoms of nausea and early satiety by impeding gastric emptying. In their landmark study of 24 diabetic patients with symptoms consistent with gastroparesis, Mearin and colleagues[3] identified periods of unusually prolonged and intense tonic pyloric contractions, or "pylorospasms," via endoscopic manometry, forming the basis of an emerging hypothesis that the pylorus is a potential therapeutic target in gastroparesis.

However, manometry has several limitations. Although it measures static pressure exerted over an area of surrounding tissue, it cannot quantify radial force nor can it distinguish between relaxed and contracted state.[9] Newer technologies such as the endoFLIP may overcome these issues, as first suggested by McMahon and colleagues[10] in 2007. Two studies have investigated the pyloric sphincter using this technique. The first study noted decreased pyloric compliance in patients with gastroparesis compared with healthy volunteers.[11] The second more robust study by Malik and colleagues[12] evaluated both idiopathic and diabetic gastroparesis and demonstrated an inverse correlation with diameter and cross-sectional area of the pylorus with early satiety and postprandial fullness. In addition, the basal pyloric pressure was observed to be elevated in almost half of the patients with nausea and vomiting and delayed gastric emptying. Interestingly, in contrast to the authors' hypothesis, no differences were found between idiopathic gastroparesis and diabetic gastroparesis.

It is therefore reasonable to conclude that pyloric dysfunction exists in at least a subset of patients with gastroparesis. However, the functional significance of this finding remains unknown. Intuitively, this may contribute to delayed gastric emptying; however, gastric-emptying rates do not correlate well with symptoms of gastroparesis.[13] Histologic data from patients with idiopathic gastroparesis and diabetic gastroparesis, that loss of interstitial cells of Cajal are seen in both subsets of patients as well as increased macrophage infiltration, suggest that the pathogenesis of the condition and associated symptoms may be more complex than previously thought.[14] What is called gastroparesis may indeed represent a spectrum of gastric neuromuscular disorders, only some of which are associated with delayed emptying, despite the presence of similar symptoms.[15] By extension, pyloric dysfunction may also be merely a manifestation of the disease, a confounding factor, or one of its culprits. Nonetheless, based on the speculation that pyloric dysfunction is responsible for the delay in gastric emptying seen in gastroparesis, an argument has been made to target the sphincter using BoNT injections, pyloroplasty, and pyloromyotomy,[16] as well as pyloric stenting.[17] The safety and efficacy of BoNT in gastroparesis are examined more carefully in later discussion.

THERAPEUTIC USE OF BOTULINUM TOXIN

BoNT was first suggested for therapeutic application in the early nineteenth century by German medical officer Christian Kerner, who experimented with the (as yet unidentified) toxin in animal models to demonstrate its ability to cause paralysis of the skeletal muscles and loss of parasympathetic function.[18] Produced by *Clostridium botulinum*, BoNT blocks the release of the neurotransmitter acetylcholine from the presynaptic terminal by enzymatic cleavage of the synaptosomal-associated protein 25 (SNAP-25). This interferes with synaptic vesicle-plasma membrane fusion at the neuromuscular junction in both skeletal motor endplates and in visceral organs, resulting in functional paralysis for a variable period of time typically in the range of several months.

There are 3 commercially available BoNT formulations in the United States: BOTOX (Allergan Inc, Campbell, CA, USA), Neuroblock or Myobloc (US World Meds, Louisville, KY, USA), and Dysport (Ipsen Ltd, Slough, UK). Despite being one of the most deadly neurotoxins known, the therapeutic administration of BoNT is quite safe in the miniscule dosages used clinically. A meta-analysis examining the use of BOTOX in a variety of diseases found that focal weakness at the site of the injection was the sole consistent adverse event compared with controls.[19]

Today, BoNT is widely used in a variety of neurologic, ophthalmologic, urologic, dermatologic, gastrointestinal, orthopedic, and cosmetic conditions.[20,21] Only a handful of these are approved by the Food and Drug Administration, and the rest are considered off-label use. Experimentation in spastic disorders of smooth muscle in the gastrointestinal tract was catalyzed after the toxin was first used successfully as a therapy for achalasia in 1995.[22] Subsequent applications include esophageal spasm, sphincter of Oddi dysfunction, anal fissure, anismus, gastroparesis, and more recently, obesity.[23,24]

For gastroparesis, BoNT is typically delivered endoscopically as an intrapyloric injection usually under direct visualization. A sclerotherapy needle (23 or 25 G) is advanced through the biopsy channel and typically 20 to 25 U BoNT/mL is injected into each of its 4 quadrants. Normally, patients can be discharged and diet advanced as tolerated on the same day as the procedure. An endoscopic ultrasonography-guided approach has also been described to increase precision of delivery to the pyloric sphincter.[25]

BOTULINUM TOXIN IN GASTROPARESIS: CLINICAL OUTCOMES

Several studies in human adults have been published on this topic,[26–43] 2 of which were randomized controlled trials conducted by Arts and colleagues[36] in 2007 and Friedenberg and colleagues[39] in 2008. The results of the major studies are summarized in **Table 1**. Most studies involved small samples sizes and did not evaluate pyloric function before or after the intervention. The authors discuss some highlights of these trials in later discussion.

In 2002, Ezzeddine and colleagues[26] published an open-label trial of 6 patients with diabetic gastroparesis who underwent pyloric injection of 100 U BoNT. There was an average symptom improvement of 55% at 6 weeks after the procedure. Furthermore, the average solid phase gastric-emptying study improved from 27.8% to 49% at 6 weeks. The data from this small trial showed promise as did 3 limited additional open-label prospective trials published the same year, each demonstrating clinical improvement after treatment.[26–28] Among these, Miller[28] demonstrated subjective improvement in 9 out of 10 female patients with idiopathic gastroparesis for more than 24 weeks after treatment with 80 to 100 U BoNT. Of patients in this study, 70% had improved gastric-emptying study with solids; however, no patients had improvement to liquids. Of note, half of these patients required repeat BoNT injections due to symptom recurrence, although all noted improvement after the second

Table 1
Important trials in the study of botulinum toxin for gastroparesis

Source Study	Number of Patients	Study Design	Cause of Gastroparesis	BoNT Dose (IU)	Assessment of Pyloric Function?	Subjective Outcomes	Objective Outcomes
Ezzeddine et al,[26] 2002	6	Prospective, open-label	DM	100	No	Significant improvement in symptoms at 6 wk	Significant improvement in gastric emptying at 6 wk
Miller,[28] 2002	10	Prospective, open-label	Idiopathic	80–100	No	90% patients with significant improvement in symptoms at 4 wk	70% patients demonstrated improvement in solid emptying at 4 wk, no improvement in liquids
Bromer et al,[32] 2005	63	Retrospective, open-label	Idiopathic (35), DM (26), postoperative (2)	100 or 200	No	~43% patients with improved symptoms lasting ~5 mo	Not evaluated
Arts et al,[36] 2007	23	Randomized controlled, double-blind, crossover	Idiopathic (19), DM (2), postoperative (2)	100	No	No difference	No difference
Friedenberg et al,[39] 2008	32	Randomized controlled, double-blind	DM (18), idiopathic (13), postoperative (1)	200	No	No difference	Improved gastric emptying at 4 wk
Coleski et al,[41] 2009	179	Retrospective, open-label	DM (81), idiopathic (79)	100, 150, or 200	No	~51% patients with improved symptoms at 1–4 wk	Not evaluated
Hooft et al,[43] 2014	13	Retrospective, open-label	Postoperative	100	No	Not evaluated	Improved gastric emptying in 76% patients at 4 wk

injection as well. These data were promising, while also highlighting the likelihood of the need for repeated injections if BoNT is used long term. This raises concern for the consequences of possible scarring to the pylorus, potentially worsening the pyloric dysfunction that the treatment aims to mitigate. In BoNT for achalasia, repeated injections have been shown to lead to submucosal fibrosis, rendering future surgical myotomy more difficult.[44]

Following these studies, Bromer and colleagues[32] published a single-center retrospective study in 2005 evaluating 63 patients with gastroparesis (35 idiopathic, 26 diabetic, and 2 postoperative), which at that time was the largest study to date. Pyloric BoNT injection of 100 to 200 U resulted in improved symptoms in 43% of cases; however, this benefit only lasted approximately 2 months. In addition, male gender was associated with a response to treatment, and a predominant symptom of vomiting predicted a poor response to treatment. Of note, a higher dose of BoNT injection was not associated with a positive response in this limited study. An important limitation of this study was that the subjects did not undergo gastric-emptying studies or manometry following treatment, unlike the previous smaller studies that included some form of objective measurement.

Based on the promise of these early studies, researchers designed 2 controlled studies published soon thereafter. In the first of these, 23 patients with gastroparesis (19 with idiopathic disease) underwent 2 upper endoscopies at 4-week intervals with either injection of saline or 100 U BoNT in a randomized, double-blind crossover design.[36] Perhaps somewhat surprisingly, significant improvement in symptoms using the validated Gastroparesis Cardinal Symptom Index (GCSI)[45] and gastric emptying was seen after initial injection of both saline or BoNT. The investigators therefore concluded that BoNT was not superior to placebo and suggested the occurrence of "a major placebo effect after endoscopic injection therapy." A second randomized controlled trial was designed by Friedenberg and colleagues[39] examining 32 patients with diabetic or idiopathic gastroparesis. Saline or 200 U BoNT was injected in a randomized blinded fashion, and patients were followed up after 4 weeks. As with the study performed by Arts and colleagues, this trial failed to demonstrate a difference in outcomes between placebo and injection. Interestingly, again, both placebo and injection resulted in improvements in GCSI; however, only BoNT appeared to cause significant improvement in gastric emptying. Interestingly, again, both placebo and BoNT injection resulted in improvements in GCSI. However, only BoNT appeared to cause significant improvement in gastric emptying, implying that the BoNT injections may have had the desired physiological effect. The fact that it was no different than placebo clinically also emphasizes again the discrepancy between gastric emptying and symptoms. This study was limited by low statistical power (it was based on an assumption of 80% response rate), but nonetheless, coupled with the other randomized controlled trial, its results discouraged further routine use of BoNT in gastroparesis. Of note, both randomized controlled trials enrolled a heterogenous gastroparesis population, which may also potentially represent a confounding factor.

In 2009, Coleski and colleagues[41] published the largest study to date on this subject, a retrospective open-label cohort of 179 patients (81 diabetic and 79 idiopathic), with a goal of elucidating factors that may enhance response to therapy. They demonstrated that a greater clinical response corresponded to higher doses of BoNT injection (200 U vs 100 U). Their analysis also suggested that patients with idiopathic gastroparesis, women, and patients aged less than 50 year old were more likely to respond to BoNT injections (this contrasted with the Bromer study demonstrating a more likely clinical response in men). Given that BoNT therapy has been shown to be no better than placebo in control studies, the interpretation of these open-label results is hazardous at best. However, this study added important data points to the conversation regarding how to potentially target subjects for a more selective future clinical trial.

In the past year, a study was published by researchers at Wake Forest on the effect of BoNT (given in 100-U doses) or pyloric balloon dilation on patients with gastroparesis who had documented normal electrogastrograms (3 cycles per minute).[42] The investigators hypothesized that the pathophysiologic mechanism of gastroparesis in these patients was pyloric dysfunction (and not a problem with stomach corpus), and therefore, these patients were an appropriately targeted patient population for this intervention. In their retrospective cohort analysis involving 33 patients (25 of whom underwent BoNT injections and 8 of whom underwent balloon dilation), 78% reported an improvement of symptoms for at least 4 weeks. Notably, the investigators did not stratify their results based on the type of pyloric therapy received, and so conclusions cannot be drawn further on the specific effect of BoNT in gastroparesis. As with other studies, these results must be viewed with caution in light of the previous randomized controlled trials.

Taken together, the studies published on BoNT in gastroparesis to date have significant limitations. As discussed, it has been argued that one reason for the failure of these studies to demonstrate a positive treatment effect is the incorrect selection of patients most likely to benefit, that is, lacking pyloric dysfunction at baseline. Neither of the 2 randomized controlled trials measured pyloric function after BoNT injection; therefore, it is unclear if BoNT truly had the anticipated physiologic effect, aside from the hypothesized clinical effect. However, at least in the trial performed by Friedenberg and colleagues,[39] BoNT improved gastric emptying compared with placebo. Technical issues may also have contributed to these results. There remains no data regarding the ideal depth and location of the injection (many endoscopists favor a 4-quadrant approach), and inadvertent diffusion of BoNT into the gastric antrum is possible. Although more technically challenging, injections directed into the pyloric channel or proximal duodenal bulb using endoscopic ultrasound (EUS) guidance may be a superior approach for this type of treatment. Perhaps most importantly, the reason this intervention may be unsuccessful is that there is no evidence of a causal relationship between pyloric dysfunction delayed emptying and the symptoms of gastroparesis. It is therefore possible that, even in patients with documented pyloric dysfunction who receive adequate BoNT injections, dysmotility in other critical regions of the gastrointestinal tract precluded a robust symptomatic response to this treatment.

SUMMARY AND FUTURE DIRECTIONS

Gastroparesis is a heterogeneous motility disorder for which a definitive cause is not identified in most patients. Although early studies regarding the use of BoNT in gastroparesis carried hope for a relatively safe and efficacious treatment modality, more rigid analyses and randomized controlled trials are unable to support its use. A systematic review of the literature published by Bai and colleagues[46] in 2010 concluded that there was no evidence to recommend BoNT injection for gastroparesis. This sentiment is echoed in the American College of Gastroenterology clinical guidelines on the management of gastroparesis published in 2012.[47] Nonetheless, BoNT is still administered at many institutions for refractory patients, underscoring both the paucity of available treatments for patients living with this disabling condition and the critical need for further larger-scale studies. A more recent review of the literature published by Ukleja and colleagues[48] in 2015 argued that given the limited treatment options, "boto:

injections can still be considered as treatment option" for patients when other therapies have failed. In addition, in patients such as lung transplant patients, whereby the possible sequelae of gastroparesis (ie, gastric reflux leading to aspiration) may lead to graft failure, it has been proposed that the benefits of this relatively benign procedure may outweigh the risks.[43]

At this time, there is no scientific evidence to support the use of BoNT in clinical practice for patients with gastroparesis. The authors think the field may benefit from further research and carefully conducted prospective clinical trials. Researchers should consider 3 important questions before "nailing the coffin shut" on BoNT in gastroparesis. First, is there a subset of patients with gastroparesis for whom this treatment would be truly beneficial, and how would one identify and target such a population? As a corollary, are endoFLIP or manometry sufficient to identify patients who may benefit, or do other patient characteristics influence their likely response, such as age, gender, or suspected cause of gastroparesis? In addition, if the clinical response to BoNT is dose dependent as has been reported, then what dosage should be considered therapeutic? Last, because accurate administration of BoNT is ultimately dependent on the skills of the endoscopist, the possibility exists that the injections do not precisely reach the pylorus. Therefore, should EUS-guided injections be used and adequate delivery of the drug be routinely quantified (eg, with preprocedure and postprocedure pyloric measurements) to determine at very least if the BoNT achieved its pharmacologic intention before assessing clinical response?

Unless further rigorous studies demonstrate its clinical efficacy, BoNT for gastroparesis may begin to fade into the background as alternative modalities emerge for refractory patients. A newer technique, gastric peroral endoscopic myotomy, or G-POEM, is an interesting approach to treatment of gastroparesis, first described by Khashab and colleagues[49] in 2013. However, this approach should also be considered highly experimental because it is based on the same fundamental presumptions that prompted the use of BoNT. It is not clear that simply having more robust ablation of the sphincter will be helpful to improve symptoms of gastroparesis if the basis of these symptoms lies elsewhere. The literature is replete with unfulfilled promises suggested by open-label studies for functional and motility bowel disorders. As discussed in this review, randomized clinical trials often fail to validate these initial findings despite the enthusiasm of the early adopters. In this regard, many valuable lessons have been learned from BoNT, and for the sake of the patients, therapies should not be offered that have not withstood the test of rigorously designed and conducted clinical trials.

It is evident that there are no easy fixes for gastroparesis and that it will remain a challenging disorder to treat. True progress will only come when the pathophysiologic basis of symptoms and the cellular and molecular pathogenesis of this condition can be confidently identified. Then, disease-modifying agents that go beyond palliative approaches can begin to be developed, and real value can be provided to long-suffering patients.

REFERENCES

1. Hasler WL, Parkman HP, Wilson LA, et al. Psychological dysfunction is associated with symptom severity but not disease etiology or degree of gastric retention in patients with gastroparesis. Am J Gastroenterol 2010;105:2357–67.

2. Parkman HP, Yates K, Hasler WL, et al. Similarities and differences between diabetic and idiopathic gastroparesis. Clin Gastroenterol Hepatol 2011;9:1056–64.

3. Mearin F, Camilleri M, Malagelada J-R. Pyloric dysfunction in diabetics with recurrent nausea and vomiting. Gastroenterology 1986;90:1919–25.
4. Feldman M, Smith HJ, Simon TR. Gastric emptying of solid radiopaque markers: studies in healthy subjects and diabetic patients. Gastroenterology 1984;87:895–902.
5. Horowitz M, Harding PE, Chatterton BE, et al. Acute and chronic effects of domperidone on gastric emptying in diabetic autonomic neuropathy. Dig Dis Sci 1985;30:1–9.
6. Loo FD, Palmer DW, Soergel KH, et al. Gastric emptying in patients with diabetes mellitus. Gastroenterology 1984;86:485–94.
7. Schade RR, Dugas MC, Lhotsky DM, et al. Effect of metoclopramide on gastric liquid emptying in patients with diabetic gastroparesis. Dig Dis Sci 1985;30:10–5.
8. Snape WJ. Metoclopramide to treat gastroparesis due to diabetes mellitus. Ann Intern Med 1982;96:444.
9. Ata-Lawenko RM, Lee YY. Emerging roles of the endolumenal functional lumen imaging probe in gastrointestinal motility disorders. J Neurogastroenterol Motil 2017;23:164–70.
10. McMahon BP, Frøkjær JB, Kunwald P, et al. The functional lumen imaging probe (FLIP) for evaluation of the esophagogastric junction. Am J Physiol Gastrointest Liver Physiol 2007;292:G377–84.
11. Gourcerol G, Tissier F, Melchior C, et al. Impaired fasting pyloric compliance in gastroparesis and the therapeutic response to pyloric dilatation. Aliment Pharmacol Ther 2014;41:360–7.
12. Malik Z, Sankineni A, Parkman HP. Assessing pyloric sphincter pathophysiology using EndoFLIP in patients with gastroparesis. Neurogastroenterol Motil 2015;27:524–31.
13. Pasricha PJ, Colvin R, Yates K, et al. Characteristics of patients with chronic unexplained nausea and vomiting and normal gastric emptying. Clin Gastroenterol Hepatol 2011;9:567–76.e1-4.
14. Grover M, Farrugia G, Lurken MS, et al. Cellular changes in diabetic and idiopathic gastroparesis. Gastroenterology 2011;140:1575–85.e8.
15. Harer KN, Pasricha PJ. Chronic unexplained nausea and vomiting or gastric neuromuscular dysfunction (GND)? An update on nomenclature, pathophysiology and treatment, and relationship to gastroparesis. Curr Treat Options Gastroenterol 2016;14:410–9.
16. Hibbard ML, Dunst CM, Swanström LL. Laparoscopic and endoscopic pyloroplasty for gastroparesis results in sustained symptom improvement. J Gastrointest Surg 2011;15:1513–9.
17. Clarke J, Sharaiha R, Kord Valeshabad A, et al. Through-the-scope transpyloric stent placement improves symptoms and gastric emptying in patients with gastroparesis. Endoscopy 2013;45:E189–90.
18. Monheit GD, Pickett A. AbobotulinumtoxinA: a 25-year history. Aesthet Surg J 2017;37:S4–11.
19. Naumann M, Jankovic J. Safety of botulinum toxin type A: a systematic review and meta-analysis. Curr Med Res Opin 2004;20:981–90.
20. Dutta SR, Passi D, Singh M, et al. Botulinum toxin the poison that heals: a brief review. Natl J Maxillofac Surg 2016;7:10–6.
21. Jankovic J. Botulinum toxin: state of the art. Mov Disord 2017;32:1131–8.
22. Pasricha PJ, Ravich WJ, Hendrix TR, et al. Intrasphincteric botulinum toxin for the treatment of achalasia. N Engl J Med 1995;332:774–8.

23. Bang CS, Baik GH, Shin IS, et al. Effect of intragastric injection of botulinum toxin A for the treatment of obesity: a meta-analysis and meta-regression. Gastrointest Endosc 2015;81:1141–9.e1-7.

24. Friedenberg F, Gollamudi S, Parkman HP. Review: the use of botulinum toxin for the treatment of gastrointestinal motility disorders. Dig Dis Sci 2004;49: 165–75.

25. Yin G, Tan W, Hu D. Endoscopic ultrasonography-guided intrapyloric injection of botulinum toxin to treat diabetic gastroparesis. Dig Endosc 2016;28:759.

26. Ezzeddine D, Jit R, Katz N, et al. Pyloric injection of botulinum toxin for treatment of diabetic gastroparesis. Gastrointest Endosc 2002;55:920–3.

27. Lacy B. Botulinum toxin for the treatment of gastroparesis: a preliminary report. Am J Gastroenterol 2002;97:1548–52.

28. Miller L. Treatment of idiopathic gastroparesis with injection of botulinum toxin into the pyloric sphincter muscle. Am J Gastroenterol 2002;97:1653–60.

29. Gupta P, Rao SSC. Attenuation of isolated pyloric pressure waves in gastroparesis in response to botulinum toxin injection: a case report. Gastrointest Endosc 2002;56:770–2.

30. Woodward MN, Spicer RD. Intrapyloric botulinum toxin injection improves gastric emptying. J Pediatr Gastroenterol Nutr 2003;37:201–2.

31. Lacy BE, Crowell MD, Schettler-Duncan A, et al. The treatment of diabetic gastroparesis with botulinum toxin injection of the pylorus. Diabetes Care 2004;27: 2341–7.

32. Bromer MQ, Friedenberg F, Miller LS, et al. Endoscopic pyloric injection of botulinum toxin A for the treatment of refractory gastroparesis. Gastrointest Endosc 2005;61:833–9.

33. Ben-Youssef R, Baron PW, Franco E, et al. Intrapyloric injection of botulinum toxin A for the treatment of persistent gastroparesis following successful pancreas transplantation. Am J Transplant 2006;6:214–8.

34. Tcherniak A, Kashtan DH, Melzer E. Successful treatment of gastroparesis following total esophagectomy using botulinum toxin. Endoscopy 2006;38:196.

35. Dumonceau J, Giostra E, Bech C, et al. Acute delayed gastric emptying after ablation of atrial fibrillation: treatment with botulinum toxin injection. Endoscopy 2006;38:543.

36. Arts J, Holvoet L, Caenepeel P, et al. Clinical trial: a randomized-controlled cross-over study of intrapyloric injection of botulinum toxin in gastroparesis. Aliment Pharmacol Ther 2007;26:1251–8.

37. Arts J, Van Gool S, Caenepeel P, et al. Influence of intrapyloric botulinum toxin injection on gastric emptying and meal-related symptoms in gastroparesis patients. Aliment Pharmacol Ther 2006;24:661–7.

38. Kent MS, Pennathur A, Fabian T, et al. A pilot study of botulinum toxin injection for the treatment of delayed gastric emptying following esophagectomy. Surg Endosc 2007;21:754–7.

39. Friedenberg FK, Palit A, Parkman HP, et al. Botulinum toxin A for the treatment of delayed gastric emptying. Am J Gastroenterol 2008;103:416–23.

40. Mirbagheri SA, Sadeghi A, Amouie M, et al. Pyloric injection of botulinum toxin for the treatment of refractory GERD accompanied with gastroparesis: a preliminary report. Dig Dis Sci 2008;53:2621–6.

41. Coleski R, Anderson MA, Hasler WL. Factors associated with symptom response to pyloric injection of botulinum toxin in a large series of gastroparesis patients. Dig Dis Sci 2009;54:2634–42.

42. Wellington J, Scott B, Kundu S, et al. Effect of endoscopic pyloric therapies for patients with nausea and vomiting and functional obstructive gastroparesis. Auton Neurosci 2017;202:56–61.
43. Hooft N, Smith M, Huang J, et al. Gastroparesis is common after lung transplantation and may be ameliorated by botulinum toxin-A injection of the pylorus. J Heart Lung Transplant 2014;33:1314–6.
44. Patti MG, Feo CV, Arcerito M, et al. The effects of previous treatment on the results of myotomy for achalasia. Gastroenterology 1998;114:A254.
45. Revicki DA, Rentz AM, Dubois D, et al. Development and validation of a patient-assessed gastroparesis symptom severity measure: the Gastroparesis Cardinal Symptom Index. Aliment Pharmacol Ther 2003;18:141–50.
46. Bai Y, Xu M-J, Yang X, et al. A systematic review on intrapyloric botulinum toxin injection for gastroparesis. Digestion 2010;81:27–34.
47. Camilleri M, Parkman HP, Shafi MA, et al. Clinical guideline: management of gastroparesis. Am J Gastroenterol 2012;108:18–37.
48. Ukleja A, Tandon K, Shah K, et al. Endoscopic botox injections in therapy of refractory gastroparesis. World J Gastrointest Endosc 2015;7:790.
49. Khashab MA, Stein E, Clarke JO, et al. Gastric peroral endoscopic myotomy for refractory gastroparesis: first human endoscopic pyloromyotomy (with video). Gastrointest Endosc 2013;78:764–8.

Stent Placement for the Treatment of Gastroparesis

Olaya I. Brewer Gutierrez, MD[a], Mouen A. Khashab, MD[b],*

KEYWORDS

- Gastroparesis • Delayed gastric emptying • Transpyloric stenting • Pylorospasm

KEY POINTS

- Gastroparesis is a complex syndrome with poorly understood underlying mechanisms.
- Pylorospasm has been described as an underlying mechanism in a subset of patients. As a result, pylorus-directed therapies have been developed and include transpyloric stenting (TPS).
- TPS may have a role in the subset of patients with gastroparesis refractory to medical therapy and with predominant symptoms of nausea/vomiting.
- TPS is considered a temporizing technique used either to treat hospitalized patients with severe gastroparesis flares or as a triage to select patients who may respond to subsequent more durable pylorus-directed therapies (eg, surgical or endoscopic pyloromyotomy).

INTRODUCTION

Gastroparesis is a syndrome of delayed gastric emptying in the absence of mechanical obstruction, and symptoms that include early satiety, postprandial fullness, nausea, vomiting, and abdominal pain.[1] It is characterized by physiologic disturbances in antral motility, increased gastric outlet resistance, and pyloric dysfunction (ie, pylorospasm).[2] First-line treatment includes dietary modifications, antiemetics, and prokinetic medications, such as metoclopramide and domperidone. These latter medications are borderline effective and possess a substantial side-effects profile. Patients refractory to medical treatment are difficult to manage and occasionally referred for surgical treatment, including gastrostomy, jejunostomy, pyloroplasty, endoscopic gastric stimulator implantation, pyloromyotomy, and gastrectomy, with

Disclosure Statement: O.I. Brewer Gutierrez: no financial or personal disclosures. M.A. Khashab: consultant and advisory board for Boston Scientific and Olympus.
^a Division of Gastroenterology and Hepatology, Johns Hopkins Hospital, Sheikh Zayed Building, 1800 Orleans Street, Suite M2058, Baltimore, MD 21287, USA; ^b Division of Gastroenterology and Hepatology, Johns Hopkins Hospital, Sheikh Zayed Building, 1800 Orleans Street, Suite 7125G, Baltimore, MD 21287, USA
* Corresponding author.
E-mail address: mkhasha1@jhmi.edu

unpredictable response as well as high morbidity. The unpredictable response to available therapies has led to the development of endoscopic therapies for the management of gastroparesis, including botulinum toxin injection, transpyloric stenting (TPS), endoscopic pyloromyotomy, percutaneous endoscopic jejunostomy, and endoscopic ultrasound-guided gastrojejunostomy.

The mechanisms underlying gastroparesis are multifactorial and not well understood. Gastric motility is complex and includes the interrelation of the smooth muscle of the gut, interstitial cells of Cajal (ICC), afferent and efferent neurons, and the sympathetic and parasympathetic nervous systems.[3] Among the functional abnormalities that have been demonstrated in a subset of gastroparetic patients, pylorospasm continues to receive special attention given its association with anatomically focused intervention. ICCs are the pacemaker of the gastrointestinal tract, regulating gastric contractions of the fundus, body, and antrum through slow-wave propagation.[4] A histologic study from biopsies of patients with refractory gastroparesis symptoms showed pyloric depletion of ICC in comparison with healthy controls. Pyloric fibrosis was also noted in a significant majority of gastroparetic patients regardless of disease cause.[3,5,6]

Antroduodenal manometry, involving placement of a pressure-sensitive catheter across the distal stomach and proximal small bowel, remains a commonly recognized option for reliable characterization of pyloric muscle activity, although the procedure can be technically challenging and is limited in its availability. Operator expertise is required because these catheters remain prone to frequent migration, decreasing the accuracy of readings that are critically dependent on position.[5,6] High-resolution manometry has also been used, but data are limited at present. The Endolumenal Functional Lumen Imaging Probe (EndoFLIP; EndoFlip, Crospon, Ireland) is a novel method to assess pyloric function. Data on this device have been mostly obtained from series of patients with achalasia. Its principle is based on the use of impedance planimetry to record cross-sectional area (CSA) and minimum diameter of any hollow structure. Moreover, it is possible to measure distensibility and compliance of any sphincter.[3] Some investigators such as Gourcerol and colleagues[7] used EndoFLip (measurements at 10, 20, 30, and 40 mL) to demonstrate that fasting pyloric compliance was altered in gastroparetic patients, and associated with delayed gastric-emptying symptoms and decreased quality of life. Moreover, pyloric dilation in gastroparesis patients resulted in increased pyloric compliance and quality-of-life score improvement. Malik and colleagues[8] also used EndoFLip (measurements at 20, 30, 40 and 50 mL) showing that early satiety and postprandial fullness were inversely correlated with diameter and CSA of the pylorus, suggesting this technique could be helpful in selecting the subset of patients with pyloric sphincter abnormalities. Snape and colleagues[9] compared the pressure of the pylorus sphincter using a water perfusion manometer and the EndoFlip (measurement at 40 mL) in known patients with delayed gastric emptying. They also reported the distensibility of the pylorus using the EndoFLip. Pressures between the manometer and the EndoFlip balloon had good correlation. A specific cutoff of distensibility has not been established but it appears that symptoms of gastroparesis appear with distensibility less than 10 mm²/mm Hg.[4]

The lack of reliable methods for identifying pylorospasm phenotype has not hindered the empiric application of anatomically focused interventions.[5,6] There are data suggesting dietary and medical treatment alone does not modify the pyloric function.[3] Also, considering that the pylorus plays a key role in gastric-emptying data indicates that distention or disruption of the pylorus, such as when using botulinum toxin or surgical pyloroplasty, can result in symptomatic improvement in patients with refractory symptoms related to gastroparesis. Limited data from single center case series by Khashab and colleagues[10] and Clark and colleagues[11] have shown that TPS improves gastroparetic symptoms in refractory cases. This article focuses on TPS for the management of refractory gastroparesis.

INDICATIONS/CONTRAINDICATIONS

There are no definite indications for the use of TPS in the management of gastroparesis, and available data are from 2 small retrospective case series. In the authors' practice, they reserve TPS for patients with severe symptoms who have failed dietary and medical therapy. Diagnosis of gastroparesis is confirmed via a 4-hour solid-phase gastric-emptying scan, and distal obstruction is excluded with endoscopy and imaging. Patients on high doses of narcotics and those with uncontrolled psychiatric disorders are excluded. Presence of more distal bowel obstruction (even if partial) is a contraindication to TPS since (1) symptoms can be the result of obstruction rather than gastroparesis and (2) stent migration can be catastrophic in such patients with need for surgical therapy to retrieve the stent or manage complications of perforation or resulting complete bowel obstruction (**Table 1**).

SURGICAL TECHNIQUE/PROCEDURE

In order to safely place a TPS, the subsequent steps need to be carefully followed.

PREOPERATIVE PLANNING

- Gastroparesis should be confirmed with a 4-hour solid gastric-emptying study performed off narcotics
- Patients are kept on a liquid diet for 48 hours before the procedure to avoid retained food residue during the procedure
- Anticoagulants and nonaspirin antiplatelet medications need to be discontinued as per society guidelines

PREPARATION AND PATIENT POSITIONING

- Obtain informed consent. Explain risks/possible complications of stent placement and endoscopic suturing
- Procedure is typically performed under general anesthesia, given potential risk of aspiration of gastric contents
- Necessary equipment and accessories:

Table 1
Indications and contraindications for transpyloric stenting

Indications	Contraindications
• Treatment of inpatients admitted with refractory severe gastroparesis symptoms and have failed dietary and medical therapies	• Patients on high-dose narcotics
• Triage to select patients who may respond to permanent therapies directed at the pylorus (surgical pyloroplasty/endoscopic pyloromyotomy)	• Patients with uncontrolled psychiatric disorders
	• Partial or complete small bowel obstruction distal to the pylorus

○ Therapeutic double channel upper gastroscope (GIF-2TH180; Olympus, Central Valley, PA, USA). Although a single-channel upper therapeutic scope can also be used to deploy the stent, the currently available Food and Drug Administration–approved suturing device is compatible only with the Olympus double channel upper therapeutic endoscope (a new version of the suturing device compatible with most gastroscopes should be available shortly in the United States).

○ Fully covered through-the-scope esophageal stent (TTS) (Niti-S esophageal stent; Taewoong Medical, Seoul, South Korea), 18 mm × 8 cm in length

○ 0.025/0.035-inch hydrophilic guidewire

○ Endoscopic suturing device and sutures (OverStitch; Apollo Endosurgery, Austin, TX, USA)

• No fluoroscopy is required for TPS

• Patient is placed in the left lateral position for the procedure

SURGICAL PROCEDURE

Step 1: Upper endoscopy is performed to rule out mechanical obstruction and suction the stomach of retained food residue

Step 2: Advance the gastroscope deeper into the duodenum and then advance a 0.025/0.035-inch guidewire to the distal duodenum under endoscopic guidance (**Fig. 1**)

Step 3: The TTS stent is advanced over the wire under endoscopic guidance (**Fig. 2**)

Step 4: The stent is pushed forward while withdrawing the gastroscope to the stomach. The endoscopic marker for the proximal end of the stent is placed approximately 2 to 3 cm proximal from the pylorus (**Fig. 3**)

Step 5: The stent is then deployed ensuring the proximal flange is positioned in the prepyloric antrum (**Figs. 4** and **5**)

Step 6: The proximal flange of the stent is then anchored to the gastric wall using endoscopic suturing. Multiple full-thickness sutures are placed to secure the stent in place and minimize the risk of migration. Suturing should not be performed along the greater curvature to avoid interference with possible future endoscopic pyloromyotomy (**Figs. 6–8**)

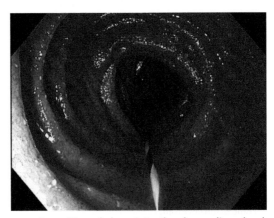

Fig. 1. The gastroscope is positioned deep into the descending duodenum and a 0.025 0.035-inch guidewire is advanced to the distal duodenum under endoscopic guidance (*Courtesy* of Boston Scientific, Marlborough, MA.)

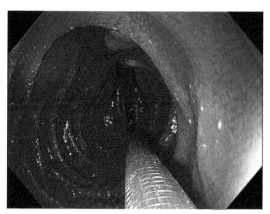

Fig. 2. The TTS stent is advanced over the wire under endoscopic guidance. (*Courtesy* of Tae-woong Medical, Gyeonggi-do, South Korea.)

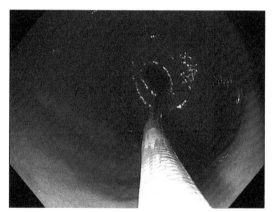

Fig. 3. The TTS is pushed forward while withdrawing the gastroscope to the stomach. The proximal stent marker is positioned 2 to 3 cm proximal from the pylorus. (*Courtesy* of Tae-woong Medical, Gyeonggi-do, South Korea.)

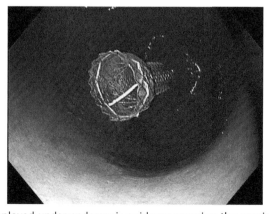

Fig. 4. Stent is deployed under endoscopic guidance ensuring the proximal flange is positioned in the prepyloric antrum. (*Courtesy* of Taewoong Medical, Gyeonggi-do, South Korea.)

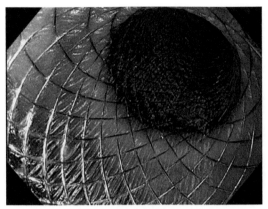

Fig. 5. Deployed stent. (*Courtesy* of Taewoong Medical, Gyeonggi-do, South Korea.)

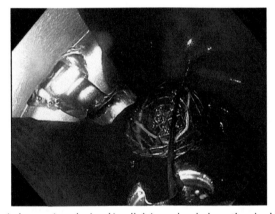

Fig. 6. The Overstitch suturing device (Apollo) is preloaded on the double channel upper endoscope (Olympus). First stitch is performed on the gastric wall. (*Courtesy* of Taewoong Medical, Gyeonggi-do, South Korea; and Apollo Endosurgery, Inc, Austin, TX; and Olympus America, Center Valley, PA.)

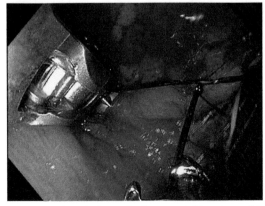

Fig. 7. The second stitch is placed through the stent. (*Courtesy* of Taewoong Medical, Gyeonggi-do, South Korea; and Apollo Endosurgery, Inc, Austin, TX; and Olympus America, Center Valley, PA.)

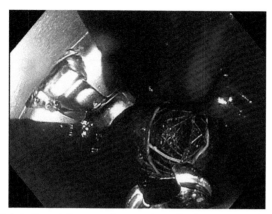

Fig. 8. A third stitch is then taken on the gastric wall. This secures the stent to the wall. (*Courtesy* of Taewoong Medical, Gyeonggi-do, South Korea; and Apollo Endosurgery, Inc, Austin, TX; and Olympus America, Center Valley, PA.)

COMPLICATIONS AND MANAGEMENT

Complications may occur during the procedure or subsequently after discharge. **Table 2** details these potential complications and their management.

POSTOPERATIVE CARE

- Patients are started on a liquid diet after the procedure. Diet may be advanced to a low-residue gastroparetic diet the following day to allow for full stent expansion
- A minority of patients will experience some degree of abdominal pain after stent insertion. This can be treated conservatively with acetaminophen or nonsteroidal

Table 2
Complications and their management

Complication	Management
Stent miss deployment/ migration	• If strong gastric contractions are observed, it is advisable to administer glucagon to inhibit gastric motility and avoid immediate stent migration after deployment • If the stent is misdeployed, the string located at the proximal flange is grasped by a large-capacity forceps. Careful pulling on the string collapses the stent for easy retrieval. If this method is not possible, then the stent is positioned in the stomach and is grasped midway along its length by the forceps. The scope and stent can then be withdrawn together • Distal stent migration should be monitored with frequent abdominal radiographs until the stent passes. The authors have occasionally retrieved migrated stents using antegrade or retrograde device-assisted enteroscopy
Duodenal perforation	• This rare complication is best treated using an over-the-scope clip whenever feasible. Failure of endoscopic closure should prompt surgical consultation • Distal stent migration may result in small bowel perforation/ obstruction. Patients should be instructed on signs and symptoms of these rare adverse events

Table 3	
Case series and retrospective study for transpyloric stenting	
Author	**Findings**
Khashab et al,[10] 2015	• 30 patients with refractory gastroparesis underwent 48 TPS procedures • 25/48 (52.1%) were performed in patients admitted to the hospital with intractable gastroparetic symptoms • Successful stent placement was achieved in 47 procedures (98%) • Clinical response was observed in 75% of patients. All inpatients were discharged • Clinical success in patients with predominant symptoms of nausea and vomiting was higher than in those with predominant symptom of pain (79% vs 21%, $P = .12$) • Stent migration was least common (48%) when stents were sutured
Clark et al,[11] 2013	• Case 1: 23-year-old woman with diabetic gastroparesis with recurrent hospitalizations. Erythromycin and metoclopramide were both unsuccessful. A 4-h solid-state gastric-emptying scintigraphy study revealed only 47% emptying at 4 h. A transpyloric stent was placed. Complete resolution of nausea and vomiting with symptoms recurrence 1 mo after procedure due to stent migration. After stent replacement, symptoms improved • Case 2: 15-year-old boy with chronic nausea and vomiting. A 4-h solid gastric scintigraphy was notable for 46% retention at 4 h. Trial of erythromycin, metoclopramide, domperidone, and promethazine was unsuccessful. He underwent transpyloric stent placement with marked clinical improvement. • Case 3: 45-year-old man with idiopathic gastroparesis. Main symptoms included early satiety and chronic nausea. A 90-min gastric-emptying study reported only 12% emptying at 90 min. Previous medical trial of erythromycin, metoclopramide, and domperidone was not successful. He underwent transpyloric stent placement with complete symptom resolution

anti-inflammatory medications. Narcotics should be avoided to circumvent worsening of gastroparetic symptoms
- Patients are followed for clinical improvement. If symptoms do not improve within 2 to 3 weeks, then the stent can be removed
- Surgical/endoscopic pyloromyotomy should be considered in patients with significant clinical improvement with TPS

OUTCOMES

There are few pieces of data published regarding TPS in the literature. A small case series and a single-center, retrospective study from the same group are presented in **Table 3**.[10,11]

SUMMARY

Gastroparesis is a complex syndrome with poorly understood underlying mechanisms. First-line treatment includes dietary medications, prokinetics, and antiemetics. When medical treatment fails, endoscopic treatment targeting the pylorus is reasonable. It is currently unknown how to best diagnose pyloric dysfunction or pylorospasm in gastroparetic patients. However, early data on EndoFLip are promising in identifying those with poor distensibility of the pylorus. TPS may have a role in the subset of patients with gastroparesis refractory to medical therapy and with predominant symptoms of nausea/vomiting. TPS can also be considered a temporizing technique used either to treat hospitalized patients with severe gastroparesis flares or as a triage to select patients who may respond to subsequent more durable pylorus-directed therapies.

REFERENCES

1. Camilleri M. Novel diet, drugs and gastric interventions for gastroparesis. Clin Gastroenterol Hepatol 2016;14:1072–80.
2. McCarty TR, Rustagi T. Endoscopic treatment of gastroparesis. World J Gastroenterol 2015;21:6842–9.
3. Clarke JO, Snape WJ Jr. Pyloric sphincter therapy: botulinum toxin, stents, and pyloromyotomy. Gastroenterol Clin North Am 2015;44:127–36.
4. Benias PC, Khashab MA. Gastric peroral endoscopic pyloromyotomy therapy for refractory gastroparesis. Curr Treat Options Gastroenterol 2017;15:637–47.
5. Ahuja NK, Clarke JO. Pyloric therapies for gastroparesis. Curr Treat Options Gastroenterol 2017;15:230–40.
6. Moraveji S, Bashashati M, Elhanafi S, et al. Depleted interstitial cells of Cajal and fibrosis in the pylorus: novel features of gastroparesis. Neurogastroenterol Motil 2016;28:1048–54.
7. Gourcerol G, Tissier F, Melchior C, et al. Impaired fasting pyloric compliance in gastroparesis and the therapeutic response to pyloric dilatation. Aliment Pharmacol Ther 2015;41:360–7.
8. Malik Z, Sankineni A, Parkman HP. Assessing pyloric sphincter pathophysiology using EndoFLIP in patients with gastroparesis. Neurogastroenterol Motil 2015;27:524–31.
9. Snape WJ, Lin MS, Agarwal N, et al. Evaluation of the pylorus with concurrent intraluminal pressure and EndoFLIP in patients with nausea and vomiting. Neurogastroenterol Motil 2016;28:758–64.
10. Khashab MA, Besharati S, Ngamruenphong S, et al. Refractory gastroparesis can be successfully managed with endoscopic transpyloric stent placement and fixation (with video). Gastrointert Endosc 2015;82:1106–9.
11. Clark JO, Sharaiha RZ, Kord Valeshabad A, et al. Through-the-scope transpylori stent placement improves symptoms and gastric emptying in patients with gastroparesis. Endoscopy 2013;45(Suppl 2 UCTN):E189–90.

Technical Aspects of Peroral Endoscopic Pyloromyotomy

Jie Tao, MD[a,b], Vaishali Patel, MD, MHS[a], Parit Mekaroonkamol, MD[a],
Hui Luo, MD[a,c], Baiwen Li, MD, PhD[a,d], Qunye Guan, MD, PhD[a,e],
Shanshan Shen, MD, PhD[a,f], Huimin Chen, MD, PhD[a,g], Qiang Cai, MD, PhD[a,h,]*

KEYWORDS

• G-POEM • Refractory gastroparesis • Technical aspects • POP

KEY POINTS

- Treatment options for gastroparesis are limited in number and efficacy. Gastric peroral endoscopic pyloromyotomy (G-POEM) has emerged as an alternate treatment option for refractory gastroparesis.
- There is no consensus regarding the technique of the G-POEM procedure.
- Identification of the pyloric muscular ring, selective circular myotomy, and a 2.5-cm to 3.0-cm length of myotomy are safe and effective.
- The optimal technique of performing G-POEM is still unknown and needs further investigation.

INTRODUCTION

Gastroparesis refers to objectively delayed gastric emptying in the absence of mechanical obstruction. It is a poorly understood, chronic, debilitating motility disorder with very limited therapeutic options.[1,2] Its prevalence has alarmingly increased

---

Disclosures: The authors have nothing to disclose.

[a] Division of Digestive Disease, Emory University School of Medicine, 1365 Clifton RD NE, Suite B 1262, Atlanta, GA 30322, USA; [b] Department of Hepatobiliary Surgery, The First Affiliated Hospital of Xi'an Jiaotong University, 227 Yanta West Road, Xi'an 710061, China; [c] Department of Pancreatobiliary Disease, Xijing Hospital of Digestive Disease, Fourth Military Medical University, 169 Changle West Road, Xi'an 710032, China; [d] Department of Gastroenterology, Shanghai General Hospital, Shanghai Jiaotong University, 100 Haining Road, Shanghai 200080, China; [e] Department of Gastroenterology, Weihai Municipal Hospital, 70 Heping Road, Weihai 264200, China; [f] Department of Gastroenterology, Nanjing Drum Tower Hospital, The Affiliated Hospital of Nanjing University Medical School, 321 Zhongshan Road, Nanjing 210008, China; [g] Department of Gastroenterology, Renji Hospital, School of Medicine, Shanghai Jiaotong University, 145 Shandongzhong Road, Shanghai 200240, China; [h] Advanced Endoscopy Fellowship, Emory University School of Medicine, 1365 Clifton Road, B1262, Atlanta, GA 30322, USA

* Corresponding author. Advanced Endoscopy Fellowship, Emory University School of Medicine, 1365 Clifton Road, B1262, Atlanta, GA 30322.

E-mail address: qcai@emory.edu

over the past decade.[3,4] Many factors have been identified as the cause of the disease, including diabetes mellitus, gastrointestinal (GI) infection, vagal nerve injury, and neurologic diseases such as multiple sclerosis; however, a significant proportion of the patients have idiopathic gastroparesis without any identifiable underlying cause.[1,5] Patients with gastroparesis suffer frequently from postprandial fullness, nausea, vomiting, bloating, and upper abdominal pain. Traditionally, gastroparesis is managed by a stepwise algorithm beginning with dietary modifications; medical therapy, including prokinetic, antiemetic, and analgesic agents; and endoscopic interventions, such as intra-pyloric botulinum injection. Surgical interventions, such as gastric electrical stimulation, laparoscopic pyloroplasty, and gastrostomy, are reserved as a last resort.[6] Furthermore, those interventions are invasive and have varying degrees of efficacy.[7–9] Surgical pyloroplasty, pyloric injection of botulinum, and placement of pylorus stents have inconsistent results.[10–12] Metoclopramide is a medication approved by the US Food and Drug Administration for gastroparesis. It has short-term effects, and its use is also associated with neurologic adverse effects. Other prokinetic agents, such as erythromycin, a macrolide antibiotic, have well-documented promotility effects but limited long-term benefit. Therefore, the treatment of gastroparesis remains quite challenging, especially for refractory cases.

Refractory gastroparesis is defined as gastroparesis confirmed by gastric emptying study (GES) and upper gastrointestinal endoscopic examination (to exclude other etiologies of nausea and vomiting) without adequate response to patients' satisfaction despite compliance to dietary modifications and a trial of maximally tolerated doses of prokinetic medications, or gastric electrical stimulator therapy. Radiologic criteria for the diagnosis of gastroparesis is a retention percentage of more than 10% at 4 hours during GES.

THE GASTRIC PERORAL ENDOSCOPIC PYLOROMYOTOMY

Peroral endoscopic myotomy (POEM) for achalasia has been in practice since 2010 and is becoming the treatment of choice for this motility disorder. Gastric peroral endoscopic pyloromyotomy (G-POEM) is a novel technique for an endoscopic incisionless pyloroplasty.[9] The principle of G-POEM is to perform myotomy at the pyloric ring using endoscopic submucosal dissection, allowing a safe and minimally invasive method of disrupting the pyloric muscle to decrease gastric outlet resistance, and thereby reduce pylorospasm.[13,14] Kawai and colleagues[15] demonstrated the feasibility of G-POEM using a live pig model. Since the first successful clinical application of the procedure in 2013,[14] subsequent small case series have demonstrated encouraging results,[16,17] and it is becoming more widely recognized as a viable therapeutic option for patients with refractory gastroparesis.[16,18,19]

In our center's previous studies, we reported the success of G-POEM for the treatment of postinfectious gastroparesis, and clinical outcomes and improvement in quality of life (QOL) after G-POEM in patients with severe refractory gastroparesis. Our results showed that G-POEM is technically safe and feasible, and effective in reducing gastroparesis symptoms and improving QOL, at least in the short-term.[19–21] Given its novelty, existing data on the procedural technique and safety are sparse, and as such there is no consensus regarding the technique.

G-POEM has surfaced as an effective, minimally invasive, alternate treatment option for refractory gastroparesis. Our high-volume center has accumulated a great deal of proficiency with this procedure, including selection of incision site, selective circular myotomy, length and depth of myotomy, identifying the pyloric muscular ring (PMR). Herein, we describe our experience with patient selection, procedural approach, and postprocedural treatment, as well as a discussion of technical aspects

PATIENT SELECTION

We carefully select patients for G-POEM from our large referral population. Patients meeting criteria for refractory gastroparesis are evaluated at our institution, and offered G-POEM based on a protocol approved by the institutional review board. We perform G-POEM in patients with significant nausea/vomiting as their predominant symptoms. Patients who have failed the gastric electrical stimulator therapy or pyloric injection of botulinum toxin are also offered the procedure. We do not routinely have an age limit, provided the patient is able to tolerate an endoscopic procedure. Exclusion criteria include patients with any contraindications to an endoscopy, inability to tolerate general anesthesia, or coagulopathy. Patients with partial gastrectomy including the antrum are also excluded. We avoid performing G-POEM on patients who are dependent on narcotics and patients who have abdominal pain as the predominant symptom (due to the concern for overlapping functional pain). Preoperative assessment of all patients includes confirmation of gastroparesis by a 4-hour GES and standard upper GI endoscopy to exclude gastric outlet obstruction.

GES is a nuclear medicine test. We usually use the solid-phase 4-hour test. At 4 hours, normal gastric retention should be less than 10%. In our experience, 80% of patients either normalize or improve their GES results after the G-POEM procedure. The average retention at 4 hours after G-POEM is approximately 20%. Gastroparesis cardinal symptom index (GCSI) is a commonly used tool for patient-reported assessment of severity of gastroparesis symptoms. GCSI is based on 3 subscales: postprandial fullness/early satiety (4 items), nausea/vomiting (3 items), and bloating (2 items) (**Table 1**).[20,22] Each subscale is graded from 0 to 5, with 5 being the most severe symptom. The average GCSI score after G-POEM is approximately 2.0.[19] Based on these values, we suggest that patients with gastric retention at 4 hours less than 20% and GCSI less than 2.5 should not be candidates for G-POEM. In other words, GES retention greater than 20% at 4 hours and GCSI greater than 2.5 should be part of the inclusion criteria.

GASTRIC PERORAL ENDOSCOPIC PYLOROMYOTOMY PROCEDURE

Patients should be kept on clear liquids for 3 days and nil per os (NPO) for 12 hours before the procedure. This 3-day preparation is a good method to avoid food retaining

Table 1
Gastroparesis Cardinal Symptom Index scores

Symptoms	None	Very Mild	Mild	Moderate	Severe	Very Severe
Nausea	0	1	2	3	4	5
Retching	0	1	2	3	4	5
Vomiting	0	1	2	3	4	5
Stomach fullness	0	1	2	3	4	5
Early satiety	0	1	2	3	4	5
Excessive postprandial fullness	0	1	2	3	4	5
Loss of appetite	0	1	2	3	4	5
Bloating	0	1	2	3	4	5
Visibly distended abdomen	0	1	2	3	4	5

in the stomach. Patients should be administered 4.5 g of piperacillin/tazobactam intravenously or 500 mg of levofloxacin intravenously (if allergic to penicillin) shortly before or during the procedure. Electrocardiogram, pulse oximetry, and blood pressure should be monitored during the procedure. All of the procedures should be performed with the patient under general anesthesia, with the patient in supine position. The stomach should be flushed with water, and the gastric residue should be removed from the gastric lumen by suctioning.

G-POEM should be started after a routine upper GI endoscopic examination. The procedure can be performed with any gastroscope with a transparent distal cap attachment. The cap not only facilitates entering the submucosal space but also can facilitate hemostasis. We usually use a hybrid I-type needle knife (ERBE, Tubingen, Germany) or a hook knife (KD-620LR; Olympus, Tokyo, Japan) for establishing a submucosal tunnel and for performing myotomy. We use carbon dioxide for insufflation during the procedure. A coag-grasper (FD-411QR; Olympus) is used to achieve hemostasis in the submucosal plane in the soft coagulation mode (ERBE) when a bleeding vessel with a diameter equal to or greater than 5 mm is encountered. The steps of G-POEM are described in our previous report.[18,20] Submucosal tunneling is performed along the posterior wall of the greater curvature of the antrum (5–6 o'clock position) using spray coagulation mode 50W on effect 2 (ERBE). Briefly, a submucosal bleb is created with a premixed methylene blue/normal saline (5 mL/500 mL) solution using a sclerotherapy needle (Olympus). A 2-cm mucosal incision is made with a hook knife or an I-type hybrid knife. A submucosal tunnel is created by dissection of submucosal fibers from the mucosal entry site to the pyloric ring. Careful attention is given to avoid any injury to the mucosal layer. An important step in performing G-POEM is maintaining the orientation toward the pyloric ring. Periodically taking the endoscope out of the submucosal tunnel and noting the bluish hue on the mucosa can ensure the correct direction of the submucosal tunnel creation. Identifying the pyloric ring is another crucial step because the duodenum can be easily damaged if submucosal dissection is extended beyond the pyloric ring. The pyloric ring is identified by direct visualization, identifying bluish color in the pylorus and in the duodenal mucosa near the pylorus. Selective circular myotomy of the pyloric circular muscle is performed and the myotomy is carefully extended for not more than 2.5 cm to 3.0 cm proximally into the antrum. After myotomy, the tunnel is rinsed with saline solution and the mucosal entry site is closed with hemostatic clips (Boston Scientific, Marlborough, MA, or Micro-Tech, Ann Arbor, MI). The process described is shown in **Fig. 1**. All material and devices used in the procedure are shown in **Table 2**. The fluoroscopy-guided method is a reliable way to identify the pyloric muscular ring[20] (**Fig. 2A**). We discuss the method later in this article.

POST GASTRIC PERORAL ENDOSCOPIC PYLOROMYOTOMY TREATMENT

All patients should be admitted to the hospital after the procedure and be kept NPO. During the NPO period, piperacillin/tazobactam or levofloxacin and a proton pump inhibitor should be administered intravenously. Patients initiate a clear liquid diet the next day if no complications have occurred after the procedure. Evaluation with an upper GI contrast study is indicated in patients with severe abdominal pain or other symptoms concerning for perforation. If no leakage is observed, then a clear liquid diet is started and advanced to soft diet as tolerated. The patients are usually discharged on the second day after the procedure with a 5-day regimen of oral amoxicillin/clavulanate or levofloxacin. Patients should be continued on proton pump inhibitor therapy for 8 weeks and longer if needed during clinical follow-up. They

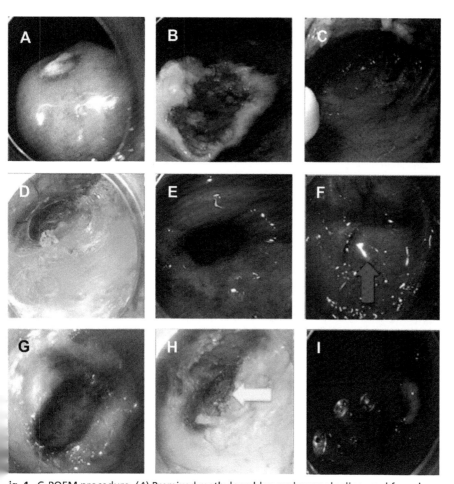

ig. 1. G-POEM procedure. (*A*) Premixed methylene blue and normal saline used for submu-
osal injection in 5 o'clock position along the greater curvature in the gastric antrum, 5 cm
roximal to the pylorus. (*B*) Mucosal incision with hybrid needle knife and creation of mu-
osotomy by lateral dissection parallel to the muscular layer to facilitate mucosal entry. (*C*)
ntry into submucosal tunnel via endoscopic submucosal dissection. Hemostasis is achieved
f apparent blood vessels with coagulation during dissection. (*D*) Creation of submucosal
unnel. (*E*) Endoscopic confirmation of extent of submucosal tunnel to the pylorus. (*F*)
he pyloric ring is identified as a thick white band (*arrow*), in contrast to a thin-walled sub-
ucosal space of the duodenum observed distally. (*G*) Pyloromyotomy is performed by
issection of the pyloric ring, exposing the muscular layer underneath. (*H*) Selective circular
yotomy approximately 2 to 3 cm in length (*arrow*). Note the arrangement of muscle fibers
erpendicular to the tunnel. (*I*) A final examination is performed to exclude mucosal injury,
nd the mucosotomy site is closed with clips.

hould maintain a soft diet for 1 week and then allowed 5 to 6 small meals of a low-
ber, low-fat diet per day.

ISCUSSIONS OF TECHNICAL ASPECTS

 number of studies have published on G-POEM treatment of refractory gastropare-
s. The studies have shown promising results, but the procedure is not widely

Table 2
Disposable materials and devices for gastric peroral endoscopy pyloromyotomy

Disposable Materials/Devices	Model
Distal cap	MH-588; Olympus, Tokyo, Japan
Injection needle	23G, NM4004–042; Olympus
Knife	Hook knife KD-620LR; Olympus Hybrid knife I-type; ERBE, Tubingen, Germany
Endoclip	Boston Scientific, Micro-Tech, Marlborough, MI
Coagulating forceps	Coagrasper, FD-411QR; Olympus
Endoscopy tower	EXERAII; Olympus
Endoscope	GIF-H190; Olympus
Electrogenerator	VIO 300D; endocut (80 W) coagulation (30 W); ERBE
CO_2 insufflator	UCR; Olympus

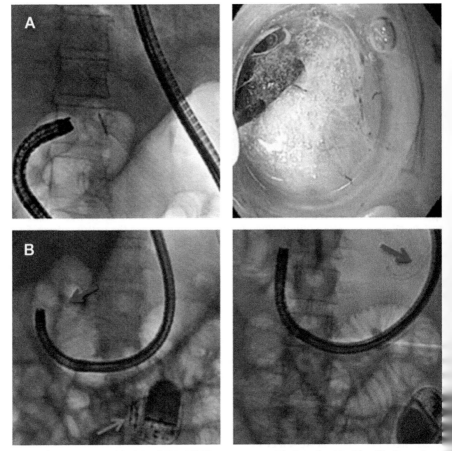

Fig. 2. Fluoroscopy-guided G-POEM. (*A*) Fluoroscopy-guided method to identify the pyloru muscular ring. (*B*) Fluoroscopic images of the gastric electrical stimulator (GES) (*blue arrow*) and its leads (*red arrow*).

available. It remains a complex procedure only performed by highly experienced endoscopists in high-volume centers. Whether the procedure can generalize with the same results if performed by less-experienced endoscopists remains questionable. Furthermore, there is also no consensus on the procedural technique. All reported studies have some technical differences, such as type of knife used for myotomy, area of mucosotomy, selective circular myotomy versus full-thickness myotomy, and the length of myotomy.[20]

Currently there is no unanimous opinion on the type of knife used for myotomy. G-POEM can be performed with different knives, such as a hook knife, hybrid knife, flush knife, dual knife, triangular-tip knife, or IT knife. The commonly used ones are hook knife (Olympus) and type I hybrid knife (ERBE). Each knife has its own advantages and disadvantages. Some investigators think a hook knife for pyloromyotomy is probably the best device for this type of procedure because of its thinness and ability to catch and resect accurately the muscular fibers of the pyloric muscle in a traction fashion due to its "hook"shape. The hybrid knife type I is stiffer and thicker than a hook knife and has a hyper pressure injection system. It cannot catch accurately fiber by fiber, and resection is performed in a pressure fashion (not the safer, traction fashion, which reduces the risk of perforation). The choice of knife should be made according to the circumstances of the procedure, such as the availability and the preference of the endoscopist.[23] Power setting is usually simple by using dry cut mode at 50 W on effect 3 (ERBE) or spray coagulation mode 50 W on effect 2 (ERBE).

Safety and operability are the main considerations for the endoscopists in selecting the site for mucosal incision. If initial mucosal incision is performed on the anterior gastric wall, the gastroscope may not be able to get into the submucosal tunnel easily because of suboptimal angulation. Of course, this procedure can be done in the anterior wall for mucosal entry, but most studies have since chosen the greater curvature or posterior gastric antral wall as the entrance site of the submucosal tunnel.

Identification of the PMR is not always easy, and can be a technical challenge during a G-POEM procedure, even for experienced hands. The submucosal tunnel at the pylorus is a narrowed space, and a landmark at this area is not always easily identified. The conventional method to facilitate identification of the PMR is taking the scope out of the submucosal tunnel and advancing it to the pylorus to observe any blue color at the pylorus or at the duodenum near the pylorus. If blue-colored mucosa is observed, it is an indication that the submucosal tunnel has reached the pylorus area and no further tunneling is necessary. Therefore, the blue-colored mucosa serves as an indirect marker of the location of the PMR. However, even if the blue-colored mucosa was observed at the pylorus and at the duodenal mucosa near the pylorus, the PMR cannot be identified in all cases. Myotomy is usually performed when blue-colored mucosa is present at the duodenal side of the pylorus regardless of whether a muscular ring structure is observed or not. At that time, if a muscular ring structure is not seen, it may indicate the tunnel does not pass the pylorus or is on the side of the pylorus. In other words, the submucosal tunnel may be terminated prematurely or ended in the wrong area, not in the pylorus. Although further tunneling or adjusting the orientation of the tunnel can be performed, it is usually very difficult to find the muscular ring structure at the last minute. Additionally, continued tunneling or changing the orientation of the tunnel in such situation may significantly increase complications, such as perforation. The injected colored solution can penetrate beyond the actual location of the end of the submucosal tunnel, therefore, observation of the blue-colored mucosa in the duodenum near the pylorus is not always a marker for accurate location of the PMR. The tip of the scope may not be located at the PMR even when blue-colored mucosa is present in the duodenum near the pylorus.

There is another way to choose to identify the PMR. We use an endoclip placed at the pylorus for identifying the PMR under fluoroscopy. Placement of an endoclip at the pylorus is the reliable method to facilitate identification of the PMR. The clip can be placed at the very beginning of the procedure before making an incision at the antrum. Under fluoroscopy, the endoclip serves as the home base, keeping the orientation of submucosal tunneling, and makes the identification of the PMR relatively easy (**Fig. 2**). The PMR was identified in all cases in our previous study.[21] A more interesting finding was that the average procedure time in the fluoroscopy-guided G-POEM was significantly shorter than that of the conventional G-POEM. Although placing an endoclip adds some time to the procedure, the endoclip makes the submucosal tunneling straighter and the PMR easier to identify, therefore reducing overall procedure time.

The fluoroscopy-guided G-POEM procedure is also useful in patients who failed treatment with a gastric electric stimulator (see **Fig. 2B**). We reported 5 patients who failed treatment of gastric electric stimulator who underwent G-POEM. Under fluoroscopy, the leads of the stimulator presented at different locations in the stomach. One lead of the stimulator in a patient was at the antrum near the incision site of the G-POEM. To visualize the stimulator and avoid cutting the stimulator lead during myotomy, the procedure should be performed under fluoroscopy unless the stimulator is removed before the procedure.[24]

We perform only selective circular myotomy from approximately 2.5 to 3.0 cm proximal to the pyloric ring to 0.5 cm distal with an intention to preserve longitudinal muscle. This is achieved by carefully examining the direction of muscle fiber during myotomy. Once a white myofascial plane is encountered and the arrangement of muscle fibers underneath changes direction, the myotomy is stopped. This is typically 0.5 cm or less in depth. In some cases of refractory gastroparesis, in which the main issue may be resolved with some increased pyloric distension, a complete myotomy of the pyloric muscle may not be required. Given the significant risks of G-POEM extending completely into the duodenal muscle, the risks of a complete myotomy may be greater than the potential benefits. Even though a full-thickness myotomy in the treatment of esophageal achalasia has shown to reduce the procedure time without increasing the procedure-related adverse events or clinical reflux complications,[25] we still performed a selective inner circular myotomy in G-POEM to ensure safety of the procedure. Selective circular myotomy versus full-thickness myotomy perhaps will be a meaningful research topic in the future.

The optimal length and depth of myotomy is also unknown currently. There are few data regarding these factors. The length of myotomy we perform at the pyloric circular muscle is approximately 2.5 to 3.0 cm and the depth is typically 0.5 cm. A new prospective ex vivo animal study on the optimal length of the myotomy during G-POEM showed that a 3-cm incision was the most appropriate for enlargement of the pylorus.[26] Submucosal dissection in the duodenal bulb is prone to perforation and bleeding because of its rich blood circulation and thin wall. Therefore, the most distal point of dissection should be cautiously terminated at approximately 0.5 cm in the postpyloric channel, trying to ensure decreasing pyloric channel pressure, expansion of pyloric outlet, and avoiding bleeding or perforation. Submucosal injection of methylene blue helps identify a demarcation between thick white pyloric band and blue submucosal plane of the duodenum, which serves as an ending landmark of the myotomy. The depth of the myotomy is not always easy to assess and is hard to control even for experienced endoscopists.

The G-POEM procedure is technically demanding and requires experienced endoscopists to perform it. The possible complications are bleeding and perforation. These complications are usually manageable during the procedure. One potential life-threatening complication is abdominal compartment syndrome secondary to pneumoperitoneum. To ensure the patients' safety, all operators should be proficient in the management of pneumoperitoneum with emergent abdominal needle decompression, in addition to other complications, such as bleeding and perforation.

Although there are more and more studies on G-POEM treatment of refractory gastroparesis published, at the present time, with only limited data from early human experience of this novel procedure, there are still many technical questions left unanswered. Many factors can affect the safety and efficacy of the procedure. We believe that G-POEM has emerged as a safe and efficacious alternate treatment for refractory gastroparesis.

SUMMARY

Gastroparesis is not an uncommon disorder. G-POEM, is a novel endoscopic therapeutic procedure, and has shown significant promise as a minimally invasive option for patients with refractory gastroparesis. We describe the technical aspects of the procedure aimed to provide direction for future operators; however, there are still many unknowns and further studies are needed to establish a standardized protocol.

REFERENCES

1. Camilleri M, Parkman HP, Shafi MA, et al. Clinical guideline: management of gastroparesis. Am J Gastroenterol 2013;108:18–37.
2. Park M-I, Camilleri M. Gastroparesis: clinical update. Am J Gastroenterol 2006; 101:1129–39.
3. Jung HK, Locke GR, Schleck CD, et al. The incidence, prevalence, and outcomes of patients with gastroparesis in Olmsted County, Minnesota, from 1996 to 2006. Gastroenterology 2009;136:1225–33.
4. Wang YR, Fisher RS, Parkman HP. Gastroparesis-related hospitalizations in the United States: trends, characteristics, and outcomes, 1995–2004. Am J Gastroenterol 2008;103:313–22.
5. Hyett B, Martinez FJ, Gill BM, et al. Delayed radionucleotide gastric emptying studies predict morbidity in diabetics with symptoms of gastroparesis. Gastroenterology 2009;137:445–52.
6. Hejazi RA, McCallum RW. Treatment of refractory gastroparesis: gastric and jejunal tubes, botox, gastric electrical stimulation, and surgery. Gastrointest Endosc Clin N Am 2009;19:73–82.
7. Hibbard ML, Dunst CM, Swanstrom LL. Laparoscopic and endoscopic pyloroplasty for gastroparesis results in sustained symptom improvement. J Gastrointest Surg 2011;15:1513–9.
8. Jones MP, Maganti K. A systematic review of surgical therapy for gastroparesis. Am J Gastroenterol 2003;98:2122–9.
9. Toro JP, Lytle NW, Patel AD, et al. Efficacy of laparoscopic pyloroplasty for the treatment of gastroparesis. J Am Coll Surg 2014;218:652–60.
10. Arts J, Holvoet L, Caenepeel P, et al. Clinical trial: a randomized-controlled crossover study of intrapyloric injection of botulinum toxin in gastroparesis. Aliment Pharmacol Ther 2007;26:1251–8.
11. Friedenberg FK, Palit A, Parkman HP, et al. Botulinum toxin A for the treatment of delayed gastric emptying. Am J Gastroenterol 2008;103:416–23.
12. Khashab MA, Besharati S, Ngamruengphong S, et al. Refractory gastroparesis can be successfully managed with endoscopic transpyloric stent placement and fixation (with video). Gastrointest Endosc 2015;82:1106–9.

13. Gonzalez J-M, Vanbiervliet G, Vitton V, et al. First European human gastric peroral endoscopic myotomy, for treatment of refractory gastroparesis. Endoscopy 2015; 47:E135.
14. Khashab MA, Stein E, Clarke JO, et al. Gastric peroral endoscopic myotomy for refractory gastroparesis: first human endoscopic pyloromyotomy (with video). Gastrointest Endosc 2013;5:764–8.
15. Kawai M, Peretta S, Burckhardt O, et al. Endoscopic pyloromyotomy: a new concept of minimally invasive surgery for pyloric stenosis. Endoscopy 2012;44: 169–73.
16. Khashab MA, Ngamruengphong S, Carr-Locke D, et al. Gastric per-oral endoscopic myotomy for refractory gastroparesis: results from the first multicenter study on endoscopic pyloromyotomy (with video). Gastrointest Endosc 2017; 85:123–8.
17. Gonzalez JM, Lestelle V, Benezech A, et al. Gastric per-oral endoscopic myotomy with antro-pyloro-myotomy in the treatment of refractory gastroparesis: clinical experience with follow-up and scintigraphic evaluation (with video). Gastrointest Endosc 2017;85:132–9.
18. Gonzalez J, Benezech A, Vitton V, et al. G-POEM with antro-pyloromyotomy for the treatment of refractory gastroparesis: mid-term follow-up and factors predicting outcome. Aliment Pharmacol Ther 2017;46:364–70.
19. Dacha S, Mekaroonkamol P, Li L, et al. Outcomes and quality-of-life assessment after gastric per-oral endoscopic pyloromyotomy (with video). Gastrointest Endosc 2017;86:282–9.
20. Mekaroonkamol P, Li L, Dacha S, et al. Gastric peroral endoscopic pyloromyotomy (G-POEM) as a salvage therapy for refractory gastroparesis: a case series of different subtypes. Neurogastroenterol Motil 2016;28:1272–7.
21. Xue HB, Fan HZ, Meng XM, et al. Fluoroscopy-guided gastric peroral endoscopic pyloromyotomy (G-POEM): a more reliable and efficient method for treatment of refractory gastroparesis. Surg Endosc 2017;31:4617–24.
22. Revicki DA, Rentz AM, Dubois D, et al. Gastroparesis Cardinal Symptom Index (GCSI): development and validation of a patient reported assessment of severity of gastroparesis symptoms. Qual Life Res 2004;13:833–44.
23. Li LY, Spandorfer R, QU CM, et al. Gastric per-oral endoscopic myotomy for refractory gastroparesis: a detailed description of the procedure, our experience, and review of the literature. Surg Endosc 2018;32(8):3421–31.
24. Koul A, Dacha S, Mekarronkamol P, et al. Fluoroscopic gastric peroral endoscopic pyloromyotomy (G-POEM) in patients with a failed gastric electrical stimulator. Gastroenterol Rep (Oxf) 2018;6(2):122–6.
25. Li QL, Chen WF, Zhou PH, et al. Peroral endoscopic myotomy for the treatment of achalasia: a clinical comparative study of endoscopic full-thickness and circular muscle myotomy. J Am Coll Surg 2013;217:442–51.
26. Jung Y, Lee J, Gromski MA, et al. Assessment of the length of myotomy in peroral endoscopic pyloromyotomy (G-POEM) using a submucosal tunnel technique (video). Surg Endosc 2015;29:2377–84.

Gastric Emptying Scintigraphy Before Gastric per Oral Endoscopic Myotomy
Imaging May Inform Treatment

Robert M. Spandorfer, MD[a], Yin Zhu, MD, PhD[b],
Parit Mekaroonkamol, MD[a], James Galt, PhD[c],
Raghuveer Halkar, MD[c], Qiang Cai, MD, PhD[a],*

KEYWORDS

- G-POEM • POP • GES • Scintigraphy • Gastroparesis • Proximal • Distal
- Pyloromyotomy

KEY POINTS

- Gastric per oral endoscopic myotomy (G-POEM) clearly and significantly reduces gastric half-emptying when measured by gastric emptying scintigraphy (GES).
- Whole stomach GES has been shown to correlate to a vast array of symptoms; however, these results have not been reliably reproducible across multiple studies.
- Using GES to measure proximal and distal GES separately may provide a better understanding of an individual's pathophysiology.
- Localized GES measurements may represent an important patient selection criterion for G-POEM.

INTRODUCTION

Gastroparesis is diagnosed by a history of typical symptoms, esophagoduodenoscopy to rule out obstruction, and gastric emptying scintigraphy (GES) to demonstrate objectively delayed gastric emptying.[1] GES involves consumption of a radiolabeled meal with imaging at set time points to determine gastric retention. In 2008, the American Neurogastroenterology and Motility Society and the Society of Nuclear Medicine

Disclosure Statement: The authors have no relationships to disclose.
[a] Division of Digestive Diseases, Emory University School of Medicine, 1365 Clifton Road, B1262, Atlanta, GA 30322, USA; [b] Department of Gastroenterology, First Affiliated Hospital of Nanchang University, No. 17 Yongwaizheng Street, Nanchang City, Jiangxi 330039, China; [c] Department of Radiology and Imaging Sciences, Emory University School of Medicine, 201 Dowman Drive, Atlanta, GA 30322, USA
* Corresponding author.
E-mail address: qcai@emory.edu

Gastrointest Endoscopy Clin N Am 29 (2019) 127–137
https://doi.org/10.1016/j.giec.2018.08.014
1052-5157/19/© 2018 Elsevier Inc. All rights reserved.

released a joint statement, standardizing the length, type of meal, and diagnostic cut-offs of GES.[2]

This standardization considers GES as a study of global gastric motility; however, gastroparesis has been shown in many studies to involve multiple different pathophysiologic mechanisms beyond just delayed emptying. These include visceral hypersensitivity, impaired fundal accommodation, fundal retention, impaired antral contractions, and pylorospasm.[3-5] Unfortunately, currently, there are not many noninvasive and reliable methods for individually measuring each of these localized dysmotilities. Some examples do exist, such as the water load test, antroduodenal or pyloric manometry, barium fluoroscopy, direct endoscopy, or wireless motility capsules that are promising. However, none of these is ideal because they are often invasive, impractical, or not completely reliable.[6,7]

Although GES is currently only used as a measure of global stomach emptying, many studies have proposed that GES may contain significantly more diagnostic information on a more localized level.[8-11] A stronger understanding of which motility patterns drive a patient's individual symptoms could provide a powerful tool in directing individualized treatment. Gastric per oral endoscopic myotomy (G-POEM) is a distally acting procedure, so it stands to reason that those patients with more distally located disease would derive the most benefit. Finding a way to identify distal retainers could perhaps represent an important step in selecting patients for G-POEM. To understand how imaging can be used to determine who will benefit most from G-POEM, this article first considers what effects G-POEM has on motility, how global GES correlates to symptoms, and how localized GES may correlate to symptoms and disease mechanisms. Then, the authors' own recent data on how GES may be used to determine which patients will have success from G-POEM is reviewed.

CHANGES FOLLOWING GASTRIC PER ORAL ENDOSCOPIC MYOTOMY

To understand how G-POEM improves symptoms in gastroparesis, the motility factors at play must be considered. Sophie Geyl and colleagues[12] explore how G-POEM affects gastric motility in their recent paper, "Peroral Endoscopic Pyloromyotomy Accelerates Gastric Emptying in Healthy Pigs: Proof of Concept." They demonstrate a significant decrease in the gastric half-emptying time ($T_{1/2}$) on GES in pigs following G-POEM. This serves to demonstrate that G-POEM has a radical impact on motility and functions in part by improving gastric emptying. Dacha and colleagues[13] demonstrate a similar phenomenon with 75% of subjects with a normalized GES following G-POEM and 25% with an improved but not normalized GES. Gonzalez and colleagues[14] showed a 69.5% normalization rate of GES following G-POEM. Khashab and colleagues[15] also found a normalization rate of 85% in their sample size. Rodriguez and colleagues[16] identified a reduction in average 4-hour retention percentage from 37.2% to 20.4%, which was statistically significant ($P = .03$). Malik and colleagues[17] showed that, of 6 post-G-POEM GES, 2 normalized, 2 improved without normalizing, 1 did not change, and 1 worsened. Overall retention percentages showed improvement on average but these differences were not significant. Across multiple studies, G-POEM has been shown to have a clear and measurable effect on gastric emptying.

The next question thus becomes, what role do these motility changes play in improving a patient's symptoms? In other words, how does GES correlate with symptoms?

THE CORRELATION BETWEEN GASTRIC EMPTYING SCINTIGRAPHY AND SYMPTOMS

Park and colleagues[18] looked at 1287 subjects with functional gastroduodenal symptoms who had undergone single-photon emission computed tomography (SPECT gastric accommodation) and GES to explore how imaging abnormalities translated to symptomatology. They found that a delayed GES correlated strongly with nausea, vomiting, abdominal discomfort, bloating, belching, and weight loss. No significant difference was seen with early satiety. They also showed that accelerated emptying correlated with abdominal discomfort when compared with normal studies.

Parkman and colleagues[19] studied a group of 198 subjects with known gastroparesis and compared their symptoms to GES data. They demonstrated that retention at 4 hours correlated significantly with severity of both early satiety and postprandial fullness.

Triadafilopoulos and colleagues[20] examined a group of subjects with dyspeptic symptoms and compared them based on their GES. They found that the only significant difference between dyspeptic subjects with normal scans and those with abnormal studies was weight loss: those with objective disease on GES lost significantly more weight. There was no significant difference between the 2 groups with regard to pain, heartburn or regurgitation, bloating, nausea, vomiting, belching, or dysphagia.

Boltin and colleagues[21] studied a group of 193 subjects who underwent GES for dyspeptic symptoms. They compared symptom rates among groups of subjects with normal, delayed, and excessively delayed $T_{1/2}$. They identified a significant correlation between the presence of nausea and vomiting and the severity of GES abnormalities.

Tseng and colleagues[22] established symptom correlations to oatmeal-based GES data in a group of 60 healthy volunteers, 30 diabetic subjects, and 30 subjects with functional dyspepsia. They found strong correlations between $T_{1/2}$ and nausea, vomiting, retching, and excessive fullness after meals. No such correlation was seen in the other Gastroparesis Cardinal Symptom Index[23] (GCSI) symptoms. They also found that retention at 1 hour correlated most strongly with nausea, vomiting, and retching, whereas retention at 3 hours correlated most strongly with a loss of appetite.

Olausson and colleagues[24] examined 115 diabetic subjects using radiopaque markers under fluoroscopy and GES. They found significant correlations between food retention and symptom severity for nausea and/or vomiting, postprandial fullness or early satiety, upper abdominal pain, and regurgitation or heartburn.

Kotani and colleagues[25] looked at gastric emptying in diabetic subjects. They did not find a significant difference in symptom scores for anorexia, nausea, vomiting, abdominal distension, early satiety, heartburn, belching, or epigastric pain between those with delayed GES and those with normal GES. They also found that changes in symptom scores for each subject did not correspond with improvements in gastric emptying after diabetic intervention.

Kawamura and colleagues[26] looked at gastroparesis in subjects with chronic hepatitis C infection and found no correlation between whole stomach retention patterns and anorexia, nausea, vomiting, abdominal distension, early satiety, heartburn, belching, or epigastric pain.

Guo and colleagues[27] examined whole stomach GES in a group of 93 subjects with functional dyspepsia and 32 healthy controls and found no significant differences in dyspepsia symptoms between those with normal and those with abnormal GES.

Stanghellini and Tack[28] demonstrated that GES abnormalities did not correlate with symptoms among subjects with functional dyspepsia and was only a nonspecific finding. They suggested that gastroparesis is only differentiated from functional dyspepsia by objective imaging findings, which are not specific or meaningful data.

These findings are summarized in **Table 1**, which clearly shows that no symptom was consistently correlated with delayed whole stomach GES. It is known that G-POEM improves or even normalizes whole stomach GES, and it has been shown to also improve gastroparesis symptoms. However, it has also been shown that whole stomach GES does not necessarily correlate reliably with symptoms. Clearly, something is missing in clinicians' understanding of gastroparesis and how treatments function.

CORRELATION BETWEEN GASTRIC EMPTYING SCINTIGRAPHY AND SYMPTOMS FOLLOWING GASTRIC PER ORAL ENDOSCOPIC MYOTOMY

This is especially true when considering G-POEM. Of particular value for understanding this procedure is the study by Gonzalez and colleagues,[14] "G-POEM with Antro-Pyloromyotomy for the Treatment of Refractory Gastroparesis: Mid-Term Follow-Up and Factors Predicting Outcome," which found that 21% of the time the postprocedural GES did not mirror clinical outcomes. This was typically seen as an improvement in GCSI, without a normalization of the scan. One case, however, was described in which there was a normalization of GES without correlated symptomatic improvement. Of note, in all of the subjects, symptom-GES discordance was from an idiopathic cause, resulting in a 43% discordance in this population. Again, this shows that understanding of GES and how it links to symptoms is incomplete.

LOCALIZED USE OF GASTRIC EMPTYING SCINTIGRAPHY

The authors propose that many of the inconsistencies of GES are because it is a measure of global stomach emptying, whereas the pathophysiology of gastroparesis is known to involve multiple factors localized to more specific regions of the stomach. The question thus becomes, how can more localized GES measurements be used to better understand patients and inform clinical decisions?

Localized Gastric Emptying Scintigraphy and the Correlation to Symptoms

Many studies have sought a correlation between gastroparesis symptoms and localized GES measurements. For instance, Orthey and colleagues[11] created a value called intragastric meal distribution (IMD), which represents a ratio of proximal radioactive counts to distal counts at any given time. IMD^0 was the IMD at the initial time point of each examination. They showed that low IMD^0 was significantly associated with severe early satiety but was not significant for other symptoms of gastroparesis.

Guo and colleagues[27] used SPECT to examine whole stomach and proximal stomach emptying. They found that nausea was correlated to delays in proximal stomach emptying. They thus suggested that patients with nausea may benefit most from promotion of proximal emptying.

Kawamura and colleagues[26] found a significant correlation between distal $T_{1/2}$ and early satiety in subjects with chronic hepatitis C complicated by gastroparesis. This correlation was not seen when looking at whole stomach or proximal stomach $T_{1/2}$. No other significant differences were identified between proximal or distal retention and anorexia, nausea, vomiting, abdominal distension, early satiety, heartburn, belching, or epigastric pain.

Finally, Gonlachanvit and colleagues[9] explored how symptom profiles varied for proximal and distal retainers. In a set of 83 subjects, they correlated symptom scores with total, proximal, and distal retention compared with healthy controls. They found

Table 1
Correlations identified between gastric emptying scintigraphy and specific symptoms

	Park et al,[18] 2017	Parkman et al,[19] 2017	Triadafilopoulos et al,[20] 2017	Boltin et al,[21] 2014	Tseng et al,[22] 2014	Olausson et al,[24] 2013	Kotani et al,[25] 2014	Kawamura et al,[26] 2012
Anorexia	—	—	—	—	*	—	x	x
Nausea	*	—	x	*	*	*	x	x
Vomiting	*	—	x	*	*	*	x	x
Retching	—	—	—	—	*	—	—	—
Bloating	*	—	x	—	*	*	—	—
Belching	*	—	x	—	—	—	x	x
Early satiety	—	*	—	—	x	*	x	x
Postprandial Fullness	x	*	—	—	*	*	—	—
Belly visibly larger	—	—	—	—	x	—	x	x
Upper Abdominal Pain	*	—	x	—	—	*	x	x
Lower Abdominal pain	—	—	—	—	—	x	—	—
Weight loss	*	—	*	—	—	—	—	—
Heartburn or regurgitation	—	—	x	—	—	*	x	x
Dysphagia	—	—	x	—	—	—	—	—

*, symptom was studied and a significant difference was identified; x, symptom was studied and no significant difference was identified.

that subjects with delayed proximal gastric emptying had significantly higher rates of vomiting, nausea, early satiety, abdominal distension, and acid regurgitation at 2 hours after meal ingestion. They did not show significant differences of rates of any symptom between distal retainers and normal controls. They also found that early proximal retainers were more likely to experience acid reflux, whereas subjects with rapid proximal emptying were more likely to experience nausea. They concluded that regurgitation is associated with enhanced fundal accommodation, whereas nausea is associated with poor fundal accommodation. Finally, they found that vomiting and early satiety were both associated with increased proximal retention at 2 hours and concluded that these symptoms are caused by impaired tonic contraction following accommodation. Overall, they determined that the proximal stomach is a more likely contributor to the symptoms of functional dyspepsia than the distal stomach.

These proximal and distal symptom correlations are summarized in **Table 2**. These studies show that GES may offer a wealth of information beyond the global gastric retention data for which it is standardly used. By using a smaller region of interest to model more localized motility patterns, more can be learned about the dominating pathophysiological factors in play for each patient. There are limited data at this point; however, this clearly is a topic that needs to be further explored.

Localized Gastric Emptying Scintigraphy as a Proxy for Digestive Mechanisms

Although understanding how localized measurements correlate with symptoms is important, to use this information to guide therapy a stronger understanding of how to tie localized measurements to pathophysiologic mechanisms is necessary.

The demonstration by Tseng and colleagues[22] (see previous discussion) that food retention at different time points correlates with different symptoms likely hints at this idea that GES can be used to analyze different mechanisms. Retention at different time points may be a rough measure of each digestive step's effectiveness.

Another example is seen in the study by Kotani and colleagues[25] study, "Clinical Assessment of Delayed Gastric Emptying and Diabetic Complications Using Gastric Emptying Scintigraphy: Involvement of Vascular Disorder," which examines gastroparesis, gastric emptying, and the presence of vascular disease in a diabetic subject set. They found that intimal medial thickness and ankle-brachial index, 2 proxies for vascular disease burden, correlate strongly with gastric emptying. Of particular interest is that these values correlate most strongly with proximal stomach $T_{1/2}$, whereas no correlation is seen with distal stomach $T_{1/2}$. This implies that vascular disease caused by diabetes influences the mechanisms involved in proximal stomach emptying more so than distal. Therefore, proximal GES measurements may serve as a model of vascular disease burden in gastroparetic patients.

Table 2 Summary of statistically significant correlations identified between localized motility measurements and individual symptoms of gastroparesis		
Study	**Value**	**Symptom Correlation**
Orthey et al,[11] 2017	Low IMD^0	Early satiety
Guo et al,[27] 2012	Delayed proximal emptying	Nausea
Kawamura et al,[26] 2012	Increased distal $T_{1/2}$	Early satiety
Gonlachanvit et al,[9] 2006	Delayed proximal $T_{1/2}$	Vomiting, nausea, early satiety, abdominal distension, and acid regurgitation

Orthey and colleagues[11] showed that IMD^0 was significantly lower in subjects with impaired fundal accommodation. This makes intuitive sense because impaired fundal accommodation leads to rapid transit to the distal stomach. They thus concluded that impaired fundal accommodation is the primary driver of early satiety (also correlated with a lower IMD^0) but may be less involved in generating other symptoms. A therapy that targets fundal accommodation would be most likely to improve early satiety by this logic. They additionally found that trained readers could reliably determine

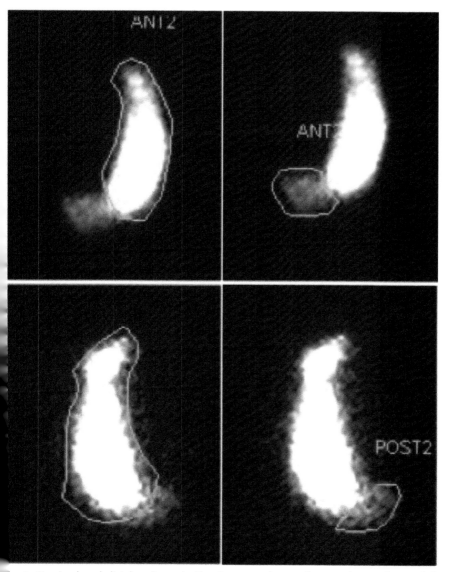

Fig. 1. Proximal and distal region selection in a sample gastric emptying study. Top-left: proximal stomach in anterior projection. Top-right: Distal stomach in anterior projection. Bottom-left: Proximal stomach in posterior projection. Bottom-right: Distal stomach in posterior projection.

whether or not there is impaired fundal accommodation for each study by simple visual inspection. Of the 99 subjects' studies they examined, 11% were ruled easy positives and 62% were easy negatives, whereas the remaining 27% were difficult or indeterminate reads. In other words, 73% of the time, the panel of readers was able to determine if impaired accommodation was present with strong reliability and consensus just by using GES, proving that this is a feasible method for measuring accommodation.

This group also examined 3 methods of defining the different regions of the stomach: (1) dividing the stomach into halves using the midpoint of the longitudinal axis of the stomach; (2) dividing the stomach into thirds along the same axis; and (3) defining proximal and distal as before or after the anatomic incisura, respectively. All 3 methods were able to differentiate normal from abnormal fundal accommodation successfully. However, the group found that the incisura was too difficult to identify in most cases.

Finally, Orthey and colleagues[11] looked at whether this new measure of fundal accommodation correlated with global GES results. They found that, of subjects with symptoms but a normal GES, 19% had an abnormally low IMD^0 value. In addition, subjects with a normal IMD^0 were more likely to have an abnormal GES than those with a low IMD^0. This demonstrates that a global GES study is only a part of the picture. Using a more localized view, significantly more clinical information can be derived, either by directly measuring a component mechanism of gastroparesis or by identifying motility issues that are missed by the whole stomach study.

LOCALIZED GASTRIC EMPTYING SCINTIGRAPHY AS A SELECTION FACTOR BEFORE GASTRIC PER ORAL ENDOSCOPIC MYOTOMY

In the authors' set of 48 subjects, we explored how GES could serve as a factor in determining who may benefit most from G-POEM. We calculated regional motility data on existing GES studies before and after G-POEM for all subjects when available. Using the incisura as an anatomic divider, the stomach was split into a proximal and distal territory. Regions of interest were drawn to delineate these areas, and localized retention percentages at 1, 2, 3, and 4 hours were calculated (**Fig. 1**). A ratio of proximal stomach $T_{1/2}$ to total stomach $T_{1/2}$ was calculated and termed the retention index

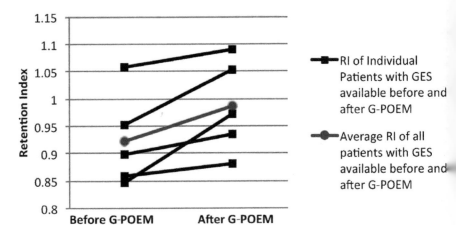

Fig. 2. Change in RI after G-POEM.

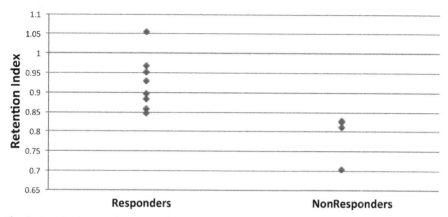

Fig. 3. Pre–G-POEM RI by responders versus nonresponders.

(RI). This was intended as a proxy for cases in which disease was localized within the stomach. A higher value indicated a relatively longer proximal $T_{1/2}$, whereas a lower value indicated a relatively shorter $T_{1/2}$ when compared with the stomach globally.

Just as the previously discussed studies demonstrated a clear reduction in $T_{1/2}$ following G-POEM, the authors also explored how G-POEM would affect motility. For all subjects in our study, there was an increase in RI, most likely due to a faster antral $T_{1/2}$ because the pyloric tone is theoretically reduced by G-POEM. The RI for the 5 subjects with both pre–G-poem and post–G-poem GES available is shown in **Fig. 2**. This represents a statistically significant increase ($P = .018$).

Responders were defined as those with a reduction in total GCSI score of 1 point, with a 25% reduction in at least 2 of 3 symptom subsets. Nonresponders and responders were grouped separately and the RI values were compared. Responders had an average RI of 0.92, whereas nonresponders averaged 0.79. This represents a statistically significant difference of 0.13 ($P<.01$). These data are demonstrated in **Fig. 3**. The authors find that, instead of a lower RI (indicating likely antral disease) predicting successful G-POEM, those with a higher RI were most likely to be responders. These preliminary results indicate that a great deal of valuable therapeutic information may be drawn from diagnostic GES. However, more research must be done to understand how to use these data effectively. The potential exists to define who will likely receive benefit from this procedure, thus decreasing unnecessary risk and maximizing therapeutic effect.

SUMMARY

GES is a powerful tool for gastroenterologists that clinicians are only beginning to understand. This article shows that G-POEM has a significant and measureable effect on GES, and that whole stomach GES does not necessarily correlate with gastroparetic symptomatology. A more localized use of GES may provide significant and valuable information about the mechanisms driving a patient's disease, and thus what type of treatment they will require. Going forward, a greater emphasis must be placed on more effectively ascertaining which disease mechanisms drive an individual patient's symptoms and how to match treatments to these more specific pathophysiologies. GES may serve as a powerful tool, not just in diagnosing gastroparesis but also in understanding what is causing retention and thus what needs to be fixed to relieve symptoms and improve quality of life.

REFERENCES

1. Stein B, Everhart KK, Lacy BE. Gastroparesis: a review of current diagnosis and treatment options. J Clin Gastroenterol 2015;49:550–8.
2. Abell TL, Camilleri M, Donohoe K, et al. Consensus recommendations for gastric emptying scintigraphy: a joint report of the American Neurogastroenterology and Motility Society and the Society of Nuclear Medicine. Am J Gastroenterol 2008; 103:753–63.
3. Maurer AH. Gastrointestinal motility, part 1: esophageal transit and gastric emptying. J Nucl Med 2015;56:1229–38.
4. Gourcerol G, Tissier F, Melchior C, et al. Impaired fasting pyloric compliance in gastroparesis and the therapeutic response to pyloric dilatation. Aliment Pharmacol Ther 2015;41:360–7.
5. Camilleri M. Novel diet, drugs, and gastric interventions for gastroparesis. Clin Gastroenterol Hepatol 2016;14:1072–80.
6. van Dyck Z, Vogele C, Blechert J, et al. The water load test as a measure of gastric interoception: development of a two-stage protocol and application to a healthy female population. PLoS One 2016;11:e0163574.
7. Clarke JO, Snape WJ Jr. Pyloric sphincter therapy: botulinum toxin, stents, and pyloromyotomy. Gastroenterol Clin North Am 2015;44:127–36.
8. Bennink R, Peeters M, Van den Maegdenbergh V, et al. Comparison of total and compartmental gastric emptying and antral motility between healthy men and women. Eur J Nucl Med 1998;25:1293–9.
9. Gonlachanvit S, Maurer AH, Fisher RS, et al. Regional gastric emptying abnormalities in functional dyspepsia and gastro-oesophageal reflux disease. Neurogastroenterol Motil 2006;18:894–904.
10. Jones KL, Horowitz M, Wishart MJ, et al. Relationships between gastric emptying, intragastric meal distribution and blood glucose concentrations in diabetes mellitus. J Nucl Med 1995;36(12):2220–8.
11. Orthey P, Yu D, Van Natta ML, et al. Intragastric meal distribution during gastric emptying scintigraphy for assessment of fundic accommodation: correlation with symptoms of gastroparesis. J Nucl Med 2017;59(4):691–7.
12. Geyl S, Legros R, Charissou A, et al. Peroral endoscopic pyloromyotomy accelerates gastric emptying in healthy pigs: proof of concept. Endosc Int Open 2016; 4:E796–9.
13. Dacha S, Mekaroonkamol P, Li L, et al. Outcomes and quality-of-life assessment after gastric per-oral endoscopic pyloromyotomy (with video). Gastrointest Endosc 2017;86:282–9.
14. Gonzalez JM, Benezech A, Vitton V, et al. G-POEM with antro-pyloromyotomy for the treatment of refractory gastroparesis: mid-term follow-up and factors predicting outcome. Aliment Pharmacol Ther 2017;46:364–70.
15. Khashab MA, Ngamruengphong S, Carr-Locke D, et al. Gastric per-oral endoscopic myotomy for refractory gastroparesis: results from the first multicenter study on endoscopic pyloromyotomy (with video). Gastrointest Endosc 2017; 85:123–8.
16. Rodriguez JH, Haskins IN, Strong AT, et al. Per oral endoscopic pyloromyotomy for refractory gastroparesis: initial results from a single institution. Surg Endosc 2017;31:5381–8.
17. Malik Z, Kataria R, Modayil R, et al. Gastric per oral endoscopic myotomy (G-POEM) for the treatment of refractory gastroparesis: early experience. Dig Dis Sci 2018. https://doi.org/10.1007/s10620-018-4976-9.

18. Park SY, Acosta A, Camilleri M, et al. Gastric motor dysfunction in patients with functional gastroduodenal symptoms. Am J Gastroenterol 2017;112:1689–99.
19. Parkman HP, Hallinan EK, Hasler WL, et al. Early satiety and postprandial fullness in gastroparesis correlate with gastroparesis severity, gastric emptying, and water load testing. Neurogastroenterol Motil 2017;29.
20. Triadafilopoulos G, Nguyen L, Clarke JO. Patients with symptoms of delayed gastric emptying have a high prevalence of oesophageal dysmotility, irrespective of scintigraphic evidence of gastroparesis. BMJ Open Gastroenterol 2017;4: e000169.
21. Boltin D, Zvidi I, Steinmetz A, et al. Vomiting and dysphagia predict delayed gastric emptying in diabetic and nondiabetic subjects. J Diabetes Res 2014; 2014:294032.
22. Tseng PH, Wu YW, Lee YC, et al. Normal values and symptom correlation of a simplified oatmeal-based gastric emptying study in the Chinese population. J Gastroenterol Hepatol 2014;29:1873–82.
23. Revicki DA, Rentz AM, Dubois D, et al. Gastroparesis Cardinal Symptom Index (GCSI): development and validation of a patient reported assessment of severity of gastroparesis symptoms. Qual Life Res 2004;13:833–44.
24. Olausson EA, Brock C, Drewes AM, et al. Measurement of gastric emptying by radiopaque markers in patients with diabetes: correlation with scintigraphy and upper gastrointestinal symptoms. Neurogastroenterol Motil 2013;25:e224–32.
25. Kotani K, Kawabe J, Kawamura E, et al. Clinical assessment of delayed gastric emptying and diabetic complications using gastric emptying scintigraphy: involvement of vascular disorder. Clin Physiol Funct Imaging 2014;34:151–8.
26. Kawamura E, Enomoto M, Kotani K, et al. Effect of mosapride citrate on gastric emptying in interferon-induced gastroparesis. Dig Dis Sci 2012;57:1510–6.
27. Guo WJ, Yao SK, Zhang YL, et al. Relationship between symptoms and gastric emptying of solids in functional dyspepsia. J Int Med Res 2012;40:1725–34.
28. Stanghellini V, Tack J. Gastroparesis: separate entity or just a part of dyspepsia? Gut 2014;63:1972–8.

Outcomes and Future Directions of Per-Oral Endoscopic Pyloromyotomy
A View from France

Jérémie Jacques, MD[a],*, Romain Legros, MD[a],
Jacques Monteil, MD, PhD[b], Denis Sautereau, MD[a],
Guillaume Gourcerol, MD, PhD[c]

KEYWORDS

- Refractory gastroparesis • Severe gastroparesis • Gastroparesis • Gastric POEM
- Per-oral pyloromyotomy • EndoFLIP

KEY POINTS

- Endoscopic per-oral pyloromyotomy (POP) is a promising therapy for refractory gastroparesis.
- Patients with pyloric dysfunction seem to be best candidates for POP.
- The Endoluminal Functional Imaging Probe, EndoFLIP (Medtronic, Minneapolis, MN, USA) could be a good tool to analyze pyloric function and selection the best candidates for POP.
- Large multicenter registries and randomized controlled trials are needed to find the best place of POP in the therapeutic armamentarium for gastroparetic patients.

 Video content accompanies this article at http://www.giendo.theclinics.com/.

INTRODUCTION

Gastroparesis is a functional disorder characterized by delayed gastric emptying in the absence of mechanical obstruction, as well as a variety of other symptoms.[1]

Grant Support: None.
Disclosures: The authors have nothing to disclose linked to this study.
Specific Author Contributions: J. Jacques and R. Legros wrote the article. J. Jacques, R. Legros, J. Monteil, D. Sautereau, and G. Gourcerol drafted and revised the article. All authors approved the final article.
[a] Gastroenterology Department, Limoges University Hospital, 2 Avenue Martin Luther King, Rouen 87042, France; [b] Nuclear Medicine Department, Limoges University Hospital, 2 Avenue Martin Luther King, Limoges 87042, France; [c] Gastroenterology Department, Rouen University Hospital, 1 rue de Germont, Rouen 76038, France
* Correspondening author. service d'Hépato-gastro-entérologie, CHU Dupuytren, Limoges 87042, France.
E-mail address: jeremiejacques@gmail.com

Gastrointest Endoscopy Clin N Am 29 (2019) 139–149
https://doi.org/10.1016/j.giec.2018.08.008
1052-5157/19/© 2018 Elsevier Inc. All rights reserved.

giendo.theclinics.com

Diagnosis of gastroparesis is problematic and it has multiple causes; however, one-third of cases are idiopathic. Esophagogastric surgery and diabetes mellitus are the 2 leading causes of gastroparesis, and the physiopathology of the disease differs according to its cause. Severe gastroparesis influences the quality of life and can lead to malnutrition. In patients with chronic diabetes it can also cause severe postprandial hypoglycemia. There are few effective therapies for gastroparesis, and those that are available are supported by a low level of evidence. A controlled diet and prokinetics are the initial treatments; however, tachyphylaxis and side effects limit their use.[2] Most patients become refractory to these therapies, and no validated alternative is available. The promising results obtained in open-label trials of gastric electric stimulation, surgical pyloroplasty, botulinum toxin injection, and transpyloric stenting in severe refractory gastroparesis were not confirmed in well-designed randomized control trials.[3–9]

Clinical trials of gastroparesis treatments are hampered by the diverse etiologic factors and pathophysiologies of the disease, which include gastric arrhythmia, neuronal damage, and decreased gastric contractility.[10,11] Manometric studies and the efficacy of pyloric-targeted therapy suggest the presence of pyloric dysfunction, also known as pylorospasm, in gastroparetic patients. Approximately 50% of these patients have a high fasting pyloric tone.[12,13] This pyloric dysfunction influences gastric emptying directly and indirectly by affecting antral and duodenal motility.

Endoscopic submucosal dissection (ESD), which was developed for precancerous and superficial cancerous lesions of the stomach, has led to the development of submucosal endoscopy.[14] Submucosal tunneling led to the development of per-oral endoscopic myotomy (POEM) for achalasia, which is safe and efficacious, although its superiority to pneumatic dilation and Heller myotomy lacks strong supporting evidence.

Submucosal tunneling enables safe access to the muscle layer, which is involved in a large number of functional disorders of the foregut. Endoscopic pyloromyotomy was recently performed for the first time in the United States by Khashab and colleagues.[15]

Because of the role of pyloric dysfunction in gastroparesis and the development of submucosal endoscopy surgery, per-oral pyloromyotomy (POP), gastric POEM (G-POEM), is being used with increasing frequency to treat refractory gastroparesis. This article focuses on the technical aspects and published results (particularly in France) of G-POEM, and on the difficulty in selecting suitable patients and the issues that must be resolved before this procedure can be performed routinely.

TECHNICAL ASPECTS AND TRAINING

Development of natural orifice transluminal endoscopic surgery (NOTES) procedures, performed in the submucosal space and based on ESD and submucosal tunneling, enabled the first performance of POP in pigs in France.[16] A circular myotomy after identification of the pyloric arch using a submucosal tunnel significantly reduced the pyloric resting pressure. In the following year, in the United States, Khashab treated a young diabetic patient with severe gastroparesis suffering from severe vomiting and diabetes imbalance, leading to recurrent hospitalization.[17] A pylorospasm was suspected because transpyloric stenting led to complete resolution of the symptoms. G-POEM markedly ameliorated these symptoms. In Europe, G-POEM was first performed in France by Barthet and colleagues.[16] Due to a high level of expertise in ESD, as well as nonreimbursement for alternative therapeutic modalities, France plays a leading role in research on the efficacy and safety of POP in patients with gastroparesis.

Using POP, the pyloric ring can be accessed by a mucosal incision along the greater or lesser curvature of the stomach. In France, more than 90% of G-POEM procedures use the greater curvature approach. Although it increases the length of the tunnel and gastric loop, this approach also increases the distance between the knife (exiting at 8–6 o'clock, depending on the endoscope) and the mucosal flap, which is important for the safety of third-space procedures.

The authors generally recommend a liquid diet for 24 hours preceding the procedure, to avoid persistence of bezoars in the gastric lumen and to decrease the risk of aspiration during anesthesia induction. POP is performed under general anesthesia with endotracheal intubation due to the risk of aspiration. Carbon dioxide insufflation is mandatory. Patients are generally placed in the supine position; however, in difficult cases, we prefer a left lateral position to decrease the length of the gastric loop. We use cefazoline prophylaxis but have no supporting evidence to justify this. A classic high-definition gastroscope with a 2.8 mm working channel is generally used. In difficult cases due to a long gastric loop, pediatric therapeutic colonoscopes (Fujinon E740 TM, Tokyo, Japan and Pentax EC-3490 TFi, Tokyo, Japan) with a 3.2 mm working channel and greater stiffness have been used. A classic transparent hood with a 4 mm hole (Olympus, Tokyo, Japan; US Endoscopy, Mentor, OH, USA) is mandatory, and a VIO 300 D or VIO 3 electrosurgical system (Erbe, Tübingen, Germany) is used.

The procedure (Video 1) is initiated by injecting the Japanese glycerol mixture, which facilitates prolonged submucosal elevation, into the submucosal space, although saline with carmine was formerly used. A mucosal incision (**Fig. 1**A) is made using an Endocut current (effect, 2; section interval, 2; cut duration, 2, VIO 3, Erbe, Tubingen, Germany), generally in a longitudinal fashion (as in esophageal POEM); however, in our experience, a horizontal mucosal incision is similarly efficacious. The first submucosal dissection is technically challenging in terms of exposing the appropriate amount of submucosal space. Fibers should be cut deep and laterally enough to push the scope into the submucosal space. A swift coagulation current is used for submucosal dissection (effect, 4; power, 80 W with a type T hybrid knife (Erbe Medical, Tübingen, Germany); and effect, 4, power, 40 W with a hook knife or dual knife [Olympus]). Submucosal tunneling (**Fig. 1**B) is the easiest part of the procedure; however, in POP, submucosal tunneling is hampered by the gastric loop and the risk of deviation of the tunneling axis. Regular checking of the direction of the tunnel (**Fig. 1**C) by monitoring the blue injection in the gastric lumen is important. A high-pressure waterjet knife facilitates tunneling by decreasing the need for exchange of devices. Perforating vessels should be prophylactically coagulated during the tunneling phase to prevent postprocedural bleeding; however, slalom between several noncoagulated intact vessels can be used to decrease the risk of mucosal flap ischemia. Prophylactic coagulation of perforating vessels is performed using a soft coagulation current (effect, power 80 W) with the tip of the knife or, for large vessels, dedicated coagulation forceps. The pyloric ring (**Fig. 1**D) is recognized as a white arch in front of the tunnel. Submucosal dissection should be continued carefully on the duodenal side before myotomy. At this stage, working in a traction fashion with the knife is safer because the mucosal flap is in front of the tip of the scope (where there is danger of mucosal damage). After separating of the pyloric ring, endoscopic pyloromyotomy can begin. We prefer to use a hook knife (**Fig. 1**E) (Olympus) to accurately cut the muscular fibers of the pylorus in a traction fashion to prevent mucosal damage. Protection of the mucosal flap is key in submucosal tunneling to ensure sufficient tightness of the myotomy site, which is essential to avoid infectious complications. In most cases, complete myotomy can be performed safely until visualization of the classic pink aspect of the serosa (**Fig. 1**F). Fusion of the muscular fibers and the serosa can prevent assessment

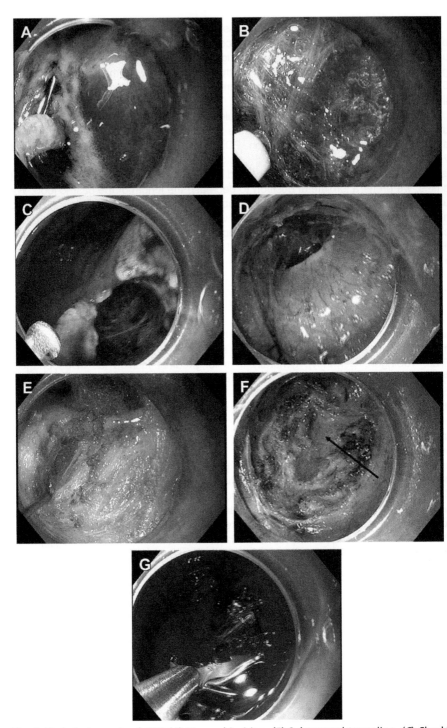

Fig. 1. Technical aspects of POP. (*A*) Mucosal incision. (*B*) Submucosal tunneling. (*C*) Check-ing the axis of the tunnel. (*D*) Identification of the pyloric ring. (*E*) Pyloromyotomy. (*F*) Com-plete myotomy with identification of the pink serosa (*arrow*). (*G*) Clip closure of the entry of the tunnel.

of the completeness of the myotomy without punctiform perforation, which did not have any clinical significance in our experience. Myotomy is generally extended by 1 to 2 cm on the antral wall.

In France, the mucosal entry site is closed using classic hemoclips (**Fig. 1**G) because endoscopic suturing is not covered by medical insurance. Two clips should be placed 5 mm distally and proximally to the end of the incision to bring and evert the edges of the mucosal incision to facilitate endoscopic closure of the mucosal entry of the tunnel.

In the Limoges Gastroenterology Department, patients fast on the day of the procedure. A liquid diet is initiated on postoperative day 1, smooth feeding on day 2, and normal feeding from day 3. Patients are usually discharged on postoperative day 2. If a perforation occurs, a nasogastric tube is inserted at the end of the procedure. The patient is required to fast for 2 days before refeeding if no pain or fever is present. On the first day of refeeding, the nasogastric tube is left in place but is clamped. If periprocedural perforation occurs, a 5-day course of amoxicillin and clavulanic acid is prescribed.

The training required to perform G-POEM depends on the operator's experience with ESD:

- Physicians with expertise in ESD: POP is easier than colorectal or esophagogastric ESD. The operator must become familiar with the semiology of the pyloric ring and the pink serosa. Video-based training and performance of the first procedure in the presence of an expert may be sufficient to achieve this.[17] Animal training can facilitate the learning of the new semiology (pyloric ring and serosa) as reported the pig study.
- Physicians without expertise in ESD: Training in the submucosal tunneling technique using in vivo and ex vivo animal models is essential. The trainee should perform several procedures in the presence of an expert to become proficient in submucosal dissection and the new semiology. Moreover, submucosal tunneling is good preparation for submucosal endoscopy and facilitates training in the ESD of premalignant and malignant lesions.

RESULTS

Six retrospective studies[18–24] on G-POEM have been published to date, and the first prospective trial of G-POEM for refractory gastroparesis was recently reported[25] (**Table 1**).

Achieving technical success is typically not problematic. However, unlike esophageal POEM in which the extent of myotomy is easy to measure because the scope is stretched, with G-POEM the consistency in the extent of myotomy is more difficult to confirm among studies; this may influence the clinical results. The clinical success rate is 73% to 90%; however, standardization of the procedure is needed.

All but 1 study[21] used the greater curvature approach for G-POEM; the study that did not report a less-marked improvement in gastric emptying time at 4 hours (37%–20%) and a reduced extent of symptom amelioration (ie, the Gastroparesis Cardinal Symptom Index [GCSI] improved from 4.6–3.3). Whether this was due to inclusion of patients having different characteristics or to the use of the lesser curvature approach is unclear.

The definition of clinical success varies among studies, which hampers interpretation of the results. A quantitative threshold of clinical success was used in only 1 gastroparesis study (decrease in the GCSI score of >0.75 points or ≥50%). Well-designed studies that use such a threshold will likely show a lower clinical success rate.

Overall, the results with POP are promising, and this procedure considerably improves the symptoms and quality of life of patients, at least in the short-term. Gonzalez

Table 1
Results of previous published series about endoscopic per-oral pyloromyotomy in refractory gastroparesis

	Design	Number of Subjects	Technical Success	Clinical Success	GES Improvement	Adverse Events	Follow-up (mo)
Shlomovitz et al,[22] 2015 (USA)	Retrospective	7	100%	86% (6/7)	80% (4/5)	1 Bleeding	6.5
Khashab et al,[18] 2016 (USA)	Retrospective	30	100%	86% (26/30)	78% (14/17)	1 Capnoperitoneum 1 Ulcer	5.5
Gonzalez et al[19,20] 2017 (France)	Retrospective	29	100%	75% (M3) 69% (M6)	87% (20/23)	5 Pneumoperitoneum 2 Bleeding 1 Abscess 1 Stricture	10
Dacha et al,[24] 2017 (USA)	Retrospective	16	100%	81% (M6)	100% (12/12)	0	6
Rodriguez et al,[21] 2018 (USA)	Retrospective	47	100%	Significant improvement	Significant improvement	0	3
Malik et al,[23] 2018 (USA)	Retrospective	13	100%	73% (M3)	66% (4/6)	0	3
Jacques et al,[25] 2018 (France)	Prospective	20	100%	90% (M3) Improvement of Gastroparesis Cardinal Symptom Index >0.75	95% (19/20)	3 perforations without clinical significance	3

Abbreviations: GES, gastric emptying scintigraphy; M3, at 3 months; M6, at 6 months.

and colleagues[20] performed a study in France with a greater than 6-month follow-up and reported that the patients could be divided into 3 groups:

- Patients with real and long-lasting improvements
- Patients with initial improvement that was lost after 3 months
- Patients in whom the procedure lacked efficacy.

A univariate analysis showed that diabetes and female gender were risk factors for treatment failure; however, these results must be confirmed in larger multicenter studies.

In the authors' experience, the clinical success rate, defined as a 0.75-point or greater improvement in GCSI score, was 90% at 3 months[25] but approximately 50% at the 1-year follow up (Jacques J, MD, 2018, unpublished data).

G-POEM accelerates gastric emptying in more than 70% of cases, as measured by 4-hour gastric emptying scintigraphy performed according to the guideline of the American Society of Nuclear Medicine. However, symptoms of gastroparesis are not systematically linked to delayed gastric emptying.

The immediate safety profile of POP is good. In the published literature, postoperative bleeding occurred in only 2 patients, with capnoperitoneum seen in 3 patients, and pulmonary embolism in 1 patient. In the authors' experience, 3 patients suffered from punctiform perforations without the need for exsufflation of the capnoperitoneum, likely due to full-thickness myotomy.

The long-term safety profile of G-POEM, taking into account the risk of biliary reflux, should be confirmed and surveillance gastroscopy should be performed.

PATIENT SELECTION

Nonrandomized studies show POP to be a useful addition to the therapeutic armamentarium[26] for patients with gastroparesis. However, the patient groups for which this procedure is most suitable remain unclear.[27] Unlike achalasia, the pathophysiology of gastroparesis is complex; therefore, a single treatment (drug, endoscopy, or surgery) is not suitable for all patients.[28–30]

An enhanced understanding of the physiopathology of gastroparesis and a means of differentiating patients according to their physiologic dysfunction (myopathic or neuronal disease, antral hypomotility, duodenal dysmotility, gastric arrhythmia, or pylorospasm) will enable selection of suitable patients. Identification of pyloric dysfunction is important for selection of patients suitable for G-POEM.

Patients with pyloric dysfunction can be identified as follows:

- Indirect evidence: A clinical response to botulinum toxin injection or transpyloric stenting. This strategy has been used in the United States[24] and should be evaluated in well-designed clinical trials. It may be useful in patients with POP not enrolled in clinical trials.
- Direct evidence: Antroduodenal manometry is the gold standard for evaluating pyloric function and was used to diagnose pylorospasm in a considerable number of diabetic patients with gastroparesis.[12] However, this procedure is technically challenging and its availability is limited. The endoluminal functional imaging probe, EndoFLIP (Medtronic, Minneapolis, MN, USA) can be used to evaluate pyloric dysfunction.[13,31,32] The EndoFLIP probe is passed alongside the scope through the pyloric channel under endoscopic visualization by grasping, using biopsy forceps, a suture attached to the distal part of the probe. Diameter, cross-sectional area, pressure, distensibility, and compliance can be measured or

calculated by the bundled software after balloon distension for 5 or more seconds. The pyloric ring is identified using a balloon inflated to 40 or 50 mL (**Fig. 2**).

Two studies have assessed the efficacy of the pyloric EndoFLIP in gastroparesis patients. The first of these reported that gastroparetic subjects have lower pyloric distensibility at 40 mL than healthy volunteers (16.2 vs. 25.2 mm^2/mm Hg, P <.05).[13] Indeed, esophagectomy subjects typically have lower distensibility than healthy volunteers (10.9 vs. 25.2 mm^2/mm Hg). Esophagectomy subjects were included as positive controls because vagus nerve damage during surgery is associated with pylorospasm. Moreover, gastroparetic subjects with a distensibility of less than 10 mm^2/mm Hg showed a better response to pyloric dilatation than other gastroparetic subjects. Using the ninetieth percentile, the cut-off for normality was 10 mm^2/mm Hg in healthy volunteers using an EndoFLIP inflated to 40 mL. There was no correlation between the EndoFLIP results and symptoms. In contrast, the second study reported a link between the results of pyloric EndoFLIP (low distensibility, low compliance, and high pressure) and symptom severity in gastroparetic subjects.[32]

In a prospective trial,[25] all subjects benefited from EndoFLIP analysis of pyloric function before G-POEM. Indeed, a high proportion of the subjects had low distensibility. Moreover, a pyloric 50 mL distensibility index of less than 9.2 mm^2/mm Hg was associated with the clinical efficacy of G-POEM (GCSI improvement >0.75 points), with 100% specificity and 72.2% sensitivity (area under the curve 0.722, 95% CI

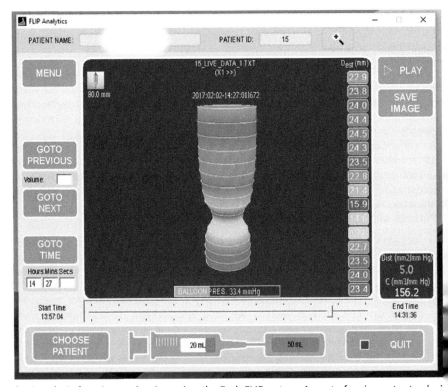

Fig. 2. Pyloric function evaluation using the EndoFLIP system. Aspect of an important pylori dysfunction with a low distensibility of the pylorus measured by an EndoFLIP probe inflated at 50 cc in a diabetic patient.

0.509–0.935; $P = .04$). The positive predictive value of this threshold was 100% but the negative predictive value was only 28.5%.

The authors' data are preliminary (obtained after 3 months of follow-up) but suggest that patients can be selected for G-POEM according to the results of pyloric function evaluation. Studies involving larger numbers of subjects and long-term follow-up are needed to confirm these results and to identify a second threshold predictive of the success or failure of G-POEM. Also, large-scale, prospective multicenter studies involving subjects with direct or indirect evidence of pyloric dysfunction are required to identify candidates for G-POEM.

FUTURE DIRECTIONS

G-POEM will likely be adopted less rapidly than esophageal POEM due to the complexity of gastroparesis. The approach, length and depth of myotomy, and the ability to repeat POP after secondary failure, should be addressed in prospective studies.

Well-designed, comparative randomized trials are needed to confirm the promising results of G-POEM, and should be designed according to Food and Drug Administration guidance for clinical evaluation of treatments for gastroparesis. Two randomized prospective studies are ongoing, 1 in France comparing (NCT02927886) G-POEM to botulinum toxin injection for refractory gastroparesis, and 1 international study comparing G-POEM to placebo with long-term follow-up (NCT03356067). These studies will pave the way for widespread use of G-POEM for gastroparesis. However, because pyloric function is not being evaluated in either of these studies, any negative results may be due to the selection of unsuitable subjects.

When in the course of gastroparesis should G-POEM be performed? Due to the low level of evidence, it is generally reserved for use in patients with severe refractory gastroparesis. However, interventions targeted at pylorospasm could alter the clinical course of gastroparesis and prevent secondary gastric dysmotility.

Combinations of treatments directed against different aspects of the pathophysiology of gastroparesis could be effective. The combination of gastric electrical stimulation and surgical pyloroplasty for severe refractory gastroparesis showed interesting results.[33] Therefore, the efficacy of the combination of endoscopic pyloromyotomy and endoscopic gastric electrical stimulation should be evaluated.

SUMMARY

POP shows promise for the treatment of gastroparesis because it improves the symptoms and quality of life of greater than 80% of patients at 3 months. However, lessons must be learned from other endoscopic therapies for pyloric dysfunction. Well-designed, randomized trials and international prospective studies with clinically relevant endpoints and evaluation of the underlying pathophysiology are required. In patients with gastroparesis, negative results in a randomized clinical trial do not necessarily signify a lack of efficacy.

POP would probably be among the most interesting therapeutic tools in the therapeutic armamentarium of physicians who take care of difficult to treat gastroparetic patients.

ACKNOWLEDGMENTS

We thanks "Protocole Hospitalier de Recherche Clinique Interrégional" for their funding for the GastroPOP trial (NCT02779920).

SUPPLEMENTARY DATA

Supplementary data related to this article can be found online at https://doi.org/10.1016/j.giec.2018.08.008.

REFERENCES

1. Camilleri M, Bharucha AE, Farrugia G. Epidemiology, mechanisms, and management of diabetic gastroparesis. Clin Gastroenterol Hepatol 2011;9(1):5–12 [quiz: e7].
2. Camilleri M, Parkman HP, Shafi MA, et al, American College of Gastroenterology. Clinical guideline: management of gastroparesis. Am J Gastroenterol 2013; 108(1):18–37 [quiz: 38].
3. Abell T, McCallum R, Hocking M, et al. Gastric electrical stimulation for medically refractory gastroparesis. Gastroenterology 2003;125(2):421–8.
4. Abell TL, Van Cutsem E, Abrahamsson H, et al. Gastric electrical stimulation in intractable symptomatic gastroparesis. Digestion 2002;66(4):204–12.
5. Gourcerol G, Huet E, Vandaele N, et al. Long term efficacy of gastric electrical stimulation in intractable nausea and vomiting. Dig Liver Dis 2012;44(7):563–8.
6. McCallum RW, Snape W, Brody F, et al. Gastric electrical stimulation with Enterra therapy improves symptoms from diabetic gastroparesis in a prospective study. Clin Gastroenterol Hepatol 2010;8(11):947–54 [quiz: e116].
7. Ahuja NK, Clarke JO. Pyloric therapies for gastroparesis. Curr Treat Options Gastroenterol 2017;15(1):230–40.
8. Bromer MQ, Friedenberg F, Miller LS, et al. Endoscopic pyloric injection of botulinum toxin A for the treatment of refractory gastroparesis. Gastrointest Endosc 2005;61(7):833–9.
9. Arts J, van Gool S, Caenepeel P, et al. Influence of intrapyloric botulinum toxin injection on gastric emptying and meal-related symptoms in gastroparesis patients. Aliment Pharmacol Ther 2006;24(4):661–7.
10. Navas CM, Patel NK, Lacy BE. Gastroparesis: medical and therapeutic advances. Dig Dis Sci 2017;62(9):2231–40.
11. Liu N, Abell T. Gastroparesis updates on pathogenesis and management. Gut Liver 2017;11(5):579–89.
12. Mearin F. Pyloric dysfunction in diabetics with recurrent nausea and vomiting. Gastroenterology 1986;90:1919–25.
13. Gourcerol G, Tissier F, Melchior C, et al. Impaired fasting pyloric compliance in gastroparesis and the therapeutic response to pyloric dilatation. Aliment Pharmacol Ther 2015;41(4):360–7.
14. Teitelbaum EN, Swanstrom LL. Submucosal surgery: novel interventions in the third space. Lancet Gastroenterol Hepatol 2017;3(2):134–40.
15. Khashab MA, Stein E, Clarke JO, et al. Gastric peroral endoscopic myotomy for refractory gastroparesis: first human endoscopic pyloromyotomy (with video). Gastrointest Endosc 2013;78(5):764–8.
16. Gonzalez J-M, Vanbiervliet G, Vitton V, et al. First European human gastric peroral endoscopic myotomy, for treatment of refractory gastroparesis. Endoscopy 2015; 47(Suppl 1 UCTN):E135–6.
17. Geyl S, Legros R, Charissou A, et al. Peroral endoscopic pyloromyotomy accelerates gastric emptying in healthy pigs: proof of concept. Endosc Int Open 2016; 4(7):E796–9.
18. Khashab MA, Ngamruengphong S, Carr-Locke D, et al. Gastric per-oral endoscopic myotomy for refractory gastroparesis: results from the first multicenter

study on endoscopic pyloromyotomy (with video). Gastrointest Endosc 2017; 85(1):123–8.

19. Gonzalez J-M, Lestelle V, Benezech A, et al. Gastric per-oral endoscopic myotomy with antropyloromyotomy in the treatment of refractory gastroparesis: clinical experience with follow-up and scintigraphic evaluation (with video). Gastrointest Endosc 2017;85(1):132–9.

20. Gonzalez JM, Benezech A, Vitton V, et al. G-POEM with antro-pyloromyotomy for the treatment of refractory gastroparesis: mid-term follow-up and factors predicting outcome. Aliment Pharmacol Ther 2017;46(3):364–70.

21. Rodriguez JH, Haskins IN, Strong AT, et al. Per oral endoscopic pyloromyotomy for refractory gastroparesis: initial results from a single institution. Surg Endosc 2018;31(12):5381–8.

22. Shlomovitz E, Pescarus R, Cassera MA, et al. Early human experience with per-oral endoscopic pyloromyotomy (POP). Surg Endosc 2015;29(3):543–51.

23. Malik Z, Kataria R, Modayil R, et al. Gastric per oral endoscopic myotomy (G-POEM) for the treatment of refractory gastroparesis: early experience. Dig Dis Sci 2018;63(9):2405–12.

24. Dacha S, Mekaroonkamol P, Li L, et al. Outcomes and quality-of-life assessment after gastric per-oral endoscopic pyloromyotomy (with video). Gastrointest Endosc 2017;86(2):282–9.

25. Jacques J, Pagnon L, Hure F, et al. Peroral endoscopic pyloromyotomy is efficacious and safe for refractory gastroparesis: prospective trial with assessment of pyloric function. Endoscopy 2018. [Epub ahead of print].

26. Camilleri M. Novel diet, drugs, and gastric interventions for gastroparesis. Clin Gastroenterol Hepatol 2016;14(8):1072–80.

27. Camilleri M, Szarka LA. POEMs for gastroparesis. Gastrointest Endosc 2017; 85(1):129–31.

28. Nguyen LA, Snape WJ. Clinical presentation and pathophysiology of gastroparesis. Gastroenterol Clin North Am 2015;44(1):21–30.

29. Parkman HP. Upper GI disorders: pathophysiology and current therapeutic approaches. Handb Exp Pharmacol 2017;239:17–37.

30. Stevens JE, Jones KL, Rayner CK, et al. Pathophysiology and pharmacotherapy of gastroparesis: current and future perspectives. Expert Opin Pharmacother 2013;14(9):1171–86.

31. Snape WJ, Lin MS, Agarwal N, et al. Evaluation of the pylorus with concurrent intraluminal pressure and EndoFLIP in patients with nausea and vomiting. Neurogastroenterol Motil 2016;28(5):758–64.

32. Malik Z, Sankineni A, Parkman HP. Assessing pyloric sphincter pathophysiology using EndoFLIP in patients with gastroparesis. Neurogastroenterol Motil 2015; 27(4):524–31.

33. Davis BR, Sarosiek I, Bashashati M, et al. The long-term efficacy and safety of pyloroplasty combined with gastric electrical stimulation therapy in gastroparesis. J Gastrointest Surg 2017;21(2):222–7.

Outcomes of Per Oral Endoscopic Pyloromyotomy in the United States

Parit Mekaroonkamol, MD, Sunil Dacha, MD,
Vaishali Patel, MD, MHS, Baiwen Li, MD, PhD, Hui Luo, MD,
Shanshan Shen, MD, PhD, Huimin Chen, MD, PhD,
Qiang Cai, MD, PhD*

KEYWORDS

- Gastroparesis • Pyloromyotomy • POP • Outcomes

KEY POINTS

- Per oral endoscopic pyloromyotomy (POP) is a safe and effective treatment for patients with refractory gastroparesis.
- Clinical outcomes of POP in the United States are promising and consistent throughout all retrospective studies and are in line with reports worldwide.
- Currently, there is no reliable predictors on clinical response to POP, although pyloric impedance planimetry appears promising as a surrogate for pyloric dysfunction.

INTRODUCTION

Per oral endoscopic pyloromyotomy (POP), also known as gastric per oral endoscopic myotomy, is a novel endoscopic intervention emerging as a new treatment for refractory gastroparesis. The procedure has gradually gained popularity due to its exciting potential in a debilitating disease whereby available therapeutic options are quite limited. This limitation is particularly true in the United States, where the incidence of gastroparesis has risen over the past decade, and only one medication, metoclopramide, is Food and Drug Administration approved for the disease.[1] Domperidone, a dopamine agonist with prokinetic activity, is also not available in the country. Despite the chronicity of gastroparesis, metoclopramide carries a black box warning of tardive dyskinesia when taken longer than 12 weeks, underscoring the need for an alternate therapy.[2]

Gastroparesis is a disease with complex pathophysiology that is yet to be fully understood. Antroduodenal hypomotility, impaired fundic accommodation, and

Disclosures: None.
Division of Digestive Diseases, Emory University School of Medicine, 615 Michael Street, Suite 201, Atlanta, GA 30322, USA
* Corresponding author.
E-mail address: qcai@emory.edu

pylorospasm are thought to play major roles in delaying gastric emptying. The physiology of gastric motility involves orchestrated interactions between each area of the stomach in a cellular level, an example of which was demonstrated by a stimulation of antroduodenal phasic motor activity by mechanically distending the gastric fundus.[3] Therefore, a mechanical disruption of the pyloric muscle may have effects beyond local pyloric dilation but rather on global gastric emptying as well. This theory was demonstrated by recent studies on surgical plyloroplasty that improved both symptoms score and gastric-emptying time.[4–7] However, it is reasonable to hypothesize that pylorus-directed therapy, such as pyloric stenting, intrapyloric botulinum injection, and POP, would be most effective in patients whose symptoms manifest from pyloric dysfunction. The challenging part is to identify those patients who would most benefit from this novel procedure.

POP uses the principle of endoscopic submucosal dissection, similar to what is used for per oral endoscopic myotomy (POEM) in achalasia, to safely identify and fully separate the pyloric ring. The procedure offers a minimally invasive and incisionless endoluminal pyloromyotomy with a comparable efficacy as its surgical counterpart, laparoscopic pyloroplasty.[8–10] Although the main concept of the procedure is the same, there are some technical variations among each center that performs POP. Clinical significance of these minor differences, such as anterior versus posterior mucosal entry, partial versus full-thickness pyloromyotomy, suturing versus endoscopic clip closure, or the use of fluoroscopy guidance to identify pyloric ring, is not yet known.[11–15] Currently, the technique performed largely depends on the endoscopist's preference. The technical details of the procedure are beyond the scope of this article.

Since its first human experience in 2013,[10] multiple centers worldwide have reported their experiences with the procedure.[8,11,12,16–21] Although early outcomes are consistently promising, generalization of these results and validation of the procedure for all gastroparesis are still premature. This article critically reviews the existing evidence regarding the outcome of POP in the United States.

INCLUSION AND EXCLUSION CRITERIA

Currently, data on clinical outcomes of POP are available from at least 7 institutions in the United States,[8,10,17,20–22] as shown in **Table 1**. Experienced endoscopists who are specialized in submucosal endoscopy are available in each center. Inclusion and exclusion criteria are almost identical across all studies and only differ in minor detail. Overall, patients who were medically refractory, defined as those who experienced ongoing symptoms despite dietary modification and maximum medical therapy, and those who could not tolerate side effects of medications were included. Diagnosis of gastroparesis was clearly established by 4-hour gastric-emptying scintigraphy (GES) or wireless motility capsule. Rodriguez and colleagues[21] were the only group who used intrapyloric botulinum injection as a preprocedure requirement to evaluate response to pylorus-directed therapy first and excluded patients who did not have clinical improvement, whereas Dacha and colleagues[17] was the only group that excluded patients with pain-predominant symptoms due to concern for overlapping functional pain. POP was performed for patients who failed the gastric electrical stimulator therapy in 2 studies.[17,20]

OUTCOME MEASUREMENTS

Clinical endpoints and follow-up duration of each study are somewhat different, as described in **Table 1**. All studies evaluated improvement in GES because it is the only objective test available in the measurement of gastric-emptying time, even

Table 1
Summary of clinical outcome of per oral endoscopic pyloromyotomy in the United States

Study	N	Cause of Gastroparesis	Outcome Measurement	Clinical Response Rate	GCSI Improvement	Improved Symptoms	GES Improvement	Adverse Event	Follow-up Period (mo)
Shlomovitz et al,[8] 2014	7	2 PSG 5 IG	• GES • Gastroparesis symptoms	85.7%	NA	• Nausea • Epigastric burning	21%–4%	1 bleeding pre-pyloric ulcer	6.5
Khashab et al,[12] 2016[a]	30	11 DG 12 PSG 7 IG	• GES • Gastroparesis symptoms	86%	NA	• Nausea • Vomiting • Abdominal pain	37%–17%	1 capnoperitonum 1 prepyloric ulcer	5.5
Dacha et al,[17] 2017	16	9 DG 1 PSG 5 IG 1 PIG	• GES • GCSI • SF-36	81%	3.4–1.5	• Nausea • Vomiting • Early satiety	62.9%–17.6%	None	12
Rodriguez et al,[21] 2017	47	12 DG 8 PSG 27 IG	• GES • GCSI	Not reported	3.6–3.3	• Nausea • Vomiting • Early satiety • Bloating	37.2%–20.4%	None	3
Malik et al,[20] 2018	11	1 DG 8 PSG 4 IG	• GES • PAGI-SYM • EndoFLIP	72.7%	2.1–1.9[c]	• Vomiting[c] • Retching[c] • Loss of appetite[c]	49%–33%[c]	1 pulmonary embolism	3

(continued on next page)

Table 1
(continued)

Study	N	Cause of Gastroparesis	Outcome Measurement	Clinical Response Rate	GCSI Improvement	Improved Symptoms	GES Improvement	Adverse Event	Follow-up Period (mo)
Mekaroonkamol et al,[27] 2018	30	12 DG 5 PSG 12 IG 1 PIG	• GES • GCSI • SF-36 • ER visit rate • Hospitalization rate	80%	3.5–2.1	• Nausea • Vomiting • Early satiety • Pain only improved up to 6 mo but not thereafter	63%–22.2%	1 tension capnoperitoneum	18
Kahaleh et al,[22] 2017[b]	33	7 DG 12 PSG 13 IG 1 Other	• GES • GCSI	85%	3.3–0.8	• Nausea • Vomiting • Early satiety • Bloating • Abdominal pain	222–143 min	1 bleeding 1 ulcer	11.5

Abbreviations: DG, diabetic gastroparesis; EndoFLIP, endoscopic functional luminal imaging probe; IG, idiopathic gastroparesis; NA, not applicable; PIG, postinfectious gastroparesis; PSG, postsurgical gastroparesis.

[a] Multicenter trial, 2 centers in the United States were involved.

[b] Abstract only publications.

[c] Not statistically significant.

though it has been shown not to correlate with clinical symptoms.[23–26] All studies evaluated postprocedure gastroparesis-related symptoms. Khashab and colleagues[12] evaluated nausea, vomiting, and abdominal pain, whereas Shlomovitz and colleagues[8] created a gastroparesis symptoms questionnaire comprising 7 symptoms that included epigastric burning and pain to evaluate symptomatic improvement. The other 5 studies used a validated scoring system, that is, Gastroparesis Cardinal Symptoms Index (GCSI), Patient Assessment of Gastrointestinal Symptoms (PAGI-SYM), and Clinical Patient Grading Assessment Score, to monitor symptoms after the procedure.[17,20–22,27] Quality of life was objectively measured in one study using a standardized short form 36 (SF-36).[17] Therefore, clinical outcomes are not completely comparable across all studies. There may be other centers that are able to offer the procedure as an alternate option for refractory gastroparesis beyond what were published in the literature, but their outcomes are not yet available to be reviewed in this article.

CLINICAL OUTCOMES OF PER ORAL ENDOSCOPIC PYLOROMYOTOMY

Among the total of 158 patients who underwent POP in the United States (this number included the multicenter study of Khashab and colleagues[12] and 2 other abstract-only publications), 68 had idiopathic gastroparesis, 47 had postsurgical gastroparesis, 43 had diabetic gastroparesis, 1 had postinfectious gastroparesis, and 1 had another cause.[8,17,20–22,27] Technical success rate was 100%, with procedural time varied from 40 to 120 minutes.[12,15,17,20,21] Overall, clinical response rate, as determined by symptomatic improvement, after POP reached 73% to 86% up to an 18-month follow-up period with low risk of major complications.[8,12,17,20,27] GCSI was the main outcome measurement in most studies.[17,20–22,27] The mean length of hospital stay was 1 to 3.3 days.[12,17,20,21] It could also improve, or even normalize, GES. However, interpretation of follow-up GES has to be performed with caution because gastric-emptying time did not always correlate well with clinical symptoms. These findings were in line with previous reposts.[17,28,29]

Significant improvement in quality of life was reported in 2 studies by the same group in the United States using the SF-36 questionnaire.[17,27] Multiple domains of various aspects in patients' quality of life, including vitality, general health, social functioning, and metal health, improved at 1 month and 6 months after the procedure. Three out of 4 domains (with the exception of general health) remained improved at 12 months. These findings were in line with a report from a European study where a mean improvement of 73% of the patients' quality of life was demonstrated after the procedure.[11] Reduction in antiemetic medication requirement and increased body weight were also demonstrated.[12,17,21]

Regarding symptoms, nausea and vomiting were consistently found to be the most responsive symptoms in all studies even though one of them did not find statistically significant improvement,[20] whereas improvement in bloating and abdominal distension was conflicting.[8,12,17,20–22,27] Most studies found no improvement in bloating subscale, with one study even showing worsened abdominal distension after POP[12,17,20,27]; however, Rodriguez and colleagues[21] and Kahaleh and colleagues[22] demonstrated improvement in bloating after POP.

Although abdominal pain is a common symptom experienced by patients with gastroparesis, it is not included in GCSI. Nevertheless, it was evaluated by most studies both directly and indirectly, using PAGI-DYM, SF-36, or direct questioning. Patients (56%–73%) reported improved abdominal pain.[12,21,22] However, the effect did not appear to sustain and lasted for only 6 months in one study.[27]

The discrepancy of these findings is still poorly understood, but it most likely can be explained by different pathophysiology of each cardinal symptom. As impaired post-prandial fundal relaxation and visceral hypersensitivity are thought to contribute to early satiety, bloating, and abdominal pain, it is thought to be less likely to respond to the POP procedure, which mainly targeted pyloric dysfunction.[30–32] On the contrary, nausea and vomiting are a result of impaired pyloric distensibility and delayed distal gastric emptying, and therefore, would be expected to respond better to the procedure.[17,33] Only the study of Dacha and colleagues[17] excluded patients with pain-predominant symptoms, but considering the conflicting results of current data and remarkable improvement in pain from Khashab and colleagues' and Rodriguez and colleagues'[21] studies, the authors believe that until more data are available, pain by itself should not be an exclusion criterion for POP. Rather, because most patients have mixed symptoms of gastroparesis, they should be advised that not all symptoms will respond equally, and the decision should be individualized.

Two failed cases underwent subsequent surgical intervention. One had laparoscopic pyloroplasty at 7 months after POP, which also did not yield any clinical response.[8] The result was not surprising because both endoscopic and laparoscopic pyloromyotomy offer the same therapeutic mechanism. The other case underwent laparoscopic total gastrectomy at 9 months after POP.[21]

One recent study by Mekaroonkamol and colleagues[27] compared the number of emergency room (ER) visits and hospitalizations related to gastroparesis 1 year before and after POP. The result showed the number of ER visits and hospitalizations related to gastroparesis significantly decreased after POP when compared with a control group in which the POP was not performed.

ADVERSE EVENTS

Overall complication rate of POP is low, ranging from 0% to 6.7%.[12,17,20–22] Serious adverse events included gastrointestinal bleed, pyloric ulcer, and tension capnoperitoneum. All bleeding during or after the procedure could be controlled endoscopically or conservatively. One case of pulmonary embolism was reported during the postprocedural recovery period.[20] The patient had a prior history of pulmonary embolism. One case of swallowing difficulty, one case of pneumonia, and one case of death not related to the procedure were reported[8,21]; otherwise, no procedure-related mortality was reported.

Despite the high rate of perforation in animal studies,[34–36] there has been no report of perforation requiring surgical intervention. This discrepancy is thought to be because of the easily distinguishable gastric circular muscle and oblique muscle in humans, as opposed to the porcine model. However, there were 2 cases of tension capnoperitoneum without frank serosal defect.[12,27] Both cases were successfully managed with intraprocedural needle percutaneous decompression, although there was no report of serious infection in the United States. There was one case of perigastric intraperitoneal abscess from a European case series.[11] It was thought to be related to diet advancement too early (the patient ate 2 hours after the procedure against medical advice). The abscess was treated conservatively with antibiotics. It is also important to acknowledge that all procedures were only performed in tertiary care centers by experts in submucosal endoscopy.

Even though the fundamental concept of POEM and POP is similar, in the authors' experience, POP is somewhat more technically challenging due to antral movement, difficulty in identifying the pyloric ring, the thin wall of the duodenum predisposing to perforation, and curvature of the prepyloric region. To minimize the risk of adverse events, it should only be performed by experienced endoscopists in high-volume centers. Its safety and efficacy profile in the community setting or academically affiliated centers remain unknown.

PREDICTIVE FACTORS

Current data of POP are still small in size and largely derived from retrospective studies, making it difficult to validate the results and generalize to clinical practice outside clinical trials. The most important question to answer is who would respond best to the procedure. Gonzalez and colleagues[11] suggested that diabetes and female gender were associated with poorer response, but this was not demonstrated in other studies.

As poor pyloric compliance and distensibility have been shown to be associated with severity of gastroparesis symptoms and delayed gastric-emptying time,[37,38] attempts to objectively identify pylorospasm using impedance planimetry technology (endoscopic functional luminal imaging probe, EndoFlip system) were made in 2 studies in the United States.[20,39] Physiologic characteristics across the pylorus, including diameter, pressure, distensibility, and cross-sectional area, were evaluated. Early satiety and postprandial fullness were inversely correlated with diameter and cross-sectional area of the pyloric sphincter.[39] These findings supported the concept of pyloromyotomy as a means to improve gastroparesis symptoms and the possibility that these pyloric measurements can serve as a predictor of clinical response to POP procedure.

Malik and colleagues[20] demonstrated that POP could decrease pyloric pressure, increase diameter and cross-sectional area, and improve pyloric distensibility and compliance immediately after endoscopic pyloromyotomy. Larger cross-sectional area after pyloromyotomy in particular was associated with reported clinical response. However, none of the preprocedure pyloric function could predict the response to the POP procedure. Although the sample size was quite small in Malik and colleagues' study, its results underscored the need to better understand the role of pyloric physiology in gastroparesis patients and the possible utility of manometric measurements in pylorus-directed therapy. Larger prospective trials are warranted to validate these results.

Rodriguez and colleagues[21] took a different approach and used clinical response to intrapyloric botulinum injection to determine candidacy to pylorus-targeted therapy with almost two-thirds of their included subjects having prior botulinum injection. Although the practice seems reasonable due to the conflicting data on efficacy of intrapyloric botulinum injection, it is probably still premature to use it as a sole inclusion criterion for the POP procedure. Perhaps future data comparing outcomes of POP between those who had prior response to botulinum injection and those who did not would be beneficial on this topic.

Because concomitant surgical pyloroplasty and gastric electrical stimulation have been shown to increase clinical benefit in gastroparesis,[5,40] perhaps POP can offer the same additional benefit. In selected patients who would benefit from gastric electrical stimulator, that is, nausea-predominant diabetic gastroparesis,[41] this should be an interesting future research topic.

Compared with outcomes reported worldwide, POP in the United States appeared to have yielded similar results in terms of efficacy and safety. In summary, POP is a minimally invasive option for treatment of refractory gastroparesis. It is technically feasible with a low risk of complications in experienced hands. At least in a midterm follow-up (up to 18 months), it has demonstrated promising efficacy in reducing gastroparesis symptoms, especially nausea/vomiting, improving quality of life, reducing health care usage, and decreasing gastric-emptying time.

However, as the field is moving forward, it is important to acknowledge that these observed benefits were derived from small retrospective studies. Although large prospective randomized trials are direly needed, the following several limitations exist: (1) Unlike POEM, there is no gold-standard intervention for gastroparesis for POP to be compared with; (2) Outcome measurements are mainly patient reported and are subject to recall bias and placebo effect; (3) GES, of which only objective testing is available at this time, does not correlate well with gastroparesis symptoms, thus cannot be used to monitor clinical response to therapy; (4) Low prevalence of gastroparesis makes it difficult to conduct a large-scale study; (5) A sham-control trial, although preferable, would be logistically difficult to conduct. Until more robust data are available, generalizability of these results remains in question.

Currently, the authors believe that POP is a viable treatment option for patients with medically refractory gastroparesis, but preferably should be performed in clinical trial settings by an experienced endoscopist and for those with nausea-predominating symptoms. Concomitant gastric electrical stimulation can be performed in selected patients with nausea-predominant diabetic gastroparesis. Pyloric and/or antroduodenal physiologic measurements, such as pyloric manometry, impedance planimetry, or wireless capsule motility, should be performed when available.

REFERENCES

1. Parkman HP, Hasler WL, Fisher RS. American Gastroenterological Association technical review on the diagnosis and treatment of gastroparesis. Gastroenterology 2004;127(5):1592–622.
2. Camilleri M, Parkman HP, Shafi MA, et al. Clinical guideline: management of gastroparesis. Am J Gastroenterol 2013;108(1):18–37.
3. Rao SS, Vemuri S, Harris B, et al. Fundic balloon distension stimulates antral and duodenal motility in man. Dig Dis Sci 2002;47(5):1015–9.
4. Davis BR, Sarosiek I, Bashashati M, et al. The long-term efficacy and safety of pyloroplasty combined with gastric electrical stimulation therapy in gastroparesis. J Gastrointest Surg 2017;21(2):222–7.
5. Sarosiek I, Forster J, Lin Z, et al. The addition of pyloroplasty as a new surgical approach to enhance effectiveness of gastric electrical stimulation therapy in patients with gastroparesis. Neurogastroenterol Motil 2013;25(2):134.
6. Hibbard ML, Dunst CM, Swanstrom LL. Laparoscopic and endoscopic pyloroplasty for gastroparesis results in sustained symptom improvement. J Gastrointest Surg 2011;15(9):1513–9.
7. Masqusi S, Velanovich V. Pyloroplasty with fundoplication in the treatment of combined gastroesophageal reflux disease and bloating. World J Surg 2007;31(2) 332–6.
8. Shlomovitz E, Pescarus R, Cassera MA, et al. Early human experience with peroral endoscopic pyloromyotomy (POP). Surg Endosc 2014;29(3):543–51.
9. Pasricha PJ, Hawari R, Ahmed I, et al. Submucosal endoscopic esophageal myotomy: a novel experimental approach for the treatment of achalasia. Gastrointest Endosc 2007;65(5):AB92.
10. Khashab MA, Stein E, Clarke JO, et al. Gastric peroral endoscopic myotomy for refractory gastroparesis: first human endoscopic pyloromyotomy (with video). Gastrointest Endosc 2013;5(78):764–8.

11. Gonzalez J, Benezech A, Vitton V, et al. G-POEM with antro-pyloromyotomy for the treatment of refractory gastroparesis: mid-term follow-up and factors predicting outcome. Aliment Pharmacol Ther 2017;46(3):364–70.
12. Khashab MA, Ngamruengphong S, Carr-Locke D, et al. Gastric per-oral endoscopic myotomy for refractory gastroparesis: results from the first multicenter study on endoscopic pyloromyotomy (with video). Gastrointest Endosc 2017; 85(1):123–8.
13. Li L, Spandorfer R, Qu C, et al. Gastric per-oral endoscopic myotomy for refractory gastroparesis: a detailed description of the procedure, our experience, and review of the literature. Surg Endosc 2018;32(8):3421–31.
14. Xue H, Fan H, Meng X, et al. Fluoroscopy-guided gastric peroral endoscopic pyloromyotomy (G-POEM): a more reliable and efficient method for treatment of refractory gastroparesis. Surg Endosc 2017;31(11):4617–24.
15. Koul A, Dacha S, Mekaroonkamol P, et al. Fluoroscopic gastric peroral endoscopic pyloromyotomy (G-POEM) in patients with a failed gastric electrical stimulator. Gastroenterol Rep (Oxf) 2018;6(2):122–6.
16. Chaves DM, de Moura EG, Mestieri LH, et al. Endoscopic pyloromyotomy via a gastric submucosal tunnel dissection for the treatment of gastroparesis after surgical vagal lesion. Gastrointest Endosc 2014;80(1):164.
17. Dacha S, Mekaroonkamol P, Li L, et al. Outcomes and quality-of-life assessment after gastric per-oral endoscopic pyloromyotomy (with video). Gastrointest Endosc 2017;86(2):282–9.
18. Jacques J, Legros R, Monteil J, et al. Gastric peroral endoscopic pyloromyotomy as a salvage therapy for refractory gastroparesis: a case series of different subtypes. Neurogastroenterol Motil 2017;29(1):e12932.
19. Mekaroonkamol P, Li L, Dacha S, et al. Gastric peroral endoscopic pyloromyotomy (G-POEM) as a salvage therapy for refractory gastroparesis: a case series of different subtypes. Neurogastroenterol Motil 2016;28(8):1272–7.
20. Malik Z, Kataria R, Modayil R, et al. Gastric per oral endoscopic myotomy (G-POEM) for the treatment of refractory gastroparesis: early experience. Dig Dis Sci 2018;63(9):2405–12.
21. Rodriguez JH, Haskins IN, Strong AT, et al. Per oral endoscopic pyloromyotomy for refractory gastroparesis: initial results from a single institution. Surg Endosc 2017;31(12):5381–8.
22. Kahaleh M, Gonzalez J-M, Baptista A, et al. 741 gastric per-oral endoscopic myotomy for the treatment of refractory gastroparesis: a multi-centered international experience. Gastrointest Endosc 2017;85(5):AB105–6.
23. Camilleri M, Szarka LA. POEMs for gastroparesis. Gastrointest Endosc 2017; 85(1):129–31.
24. Horowitz M, Harding P, Maddox A, et al. Gastric and oesophageal emptying in patients with type 2 (non-insulin-dependent) diabetes mellitus. Diabetologia 1989;32(3):151–9.
25. Horowitz M, Harding PE, Maddox A, et al. Gastric and oesophageal emptying in insulin-dependent diabetes mellitus. J Gastroenterol Hepatol 1986;1(2):97–113.
26. Khayyam U, Sachdeva P, Gomez J, et al. Assessment of symptoms during gastric emptying scintigraphy to correlate symptoms to delayed gastric emptying. Neurogastroenterol Motil 2010;22(5):539–45.
27. Mekaroonkamol P, Dacha S, Wang L, et al. Gastric peroral endoscopic pyloromyotomy reduces symptoms, increases quality of life, and reduces healthcare usage for patients with gastroparesis. Clin Gastroenterol Hepatol 2018. [Epub ahead of print].

28. Jones KL, Russo A, Stevens JE, et al. Predictors of delayed gastric emptying in diabetes. Diabetes Care 2001;24(7):1264–9.
29. Samsom M, Vermeijden J, Smout A, et al. Prevalence of delayed gastric emptying in diabetic patients and relationship to dyspeptic symptoms a prospective study in unselected diabetic patients. Diabetes Care 2003;26(11):3116–22.
30. Abell TL, Camilleri M, Donohoe K, et al. Consensus recommendations for gastric emptying scintigraphy: a joint report of the American Neurogastroenterology and Motility Society and the Society of Nuclear Medicine. Am J Gastroenterol 2008; 103(3):753–63.
31. Gonlachanvit S, Maurer A, Fisher R, et al. Regional gastric emptying abnormalities in functional dyspepsia and gastro-oesophageal reflux disease. Neurogastroenterol Motil 2006;18(10):894–904.
32. Maurer AH, Parkman HP. Update on gastrointestinal scintigraphy. Paper presented at: Seminars in nuclear medicine 2006.
33. Mekaroonkamol P, Li L, Cai Q. The role of pyloric manometry in gastric per-oral endoscopic pyloromyotomy (G-POEM): response to Jacques et al. Neurogastroenterol Motil 2017;29(1):e12949.
34. Chaves DM, Gusmon CC, Mestieri LH, et al. A new technique for performing endoscopic pyloromyotomy by gastric submucosal tunnel dissection. Surg Laparosc Endosc Percutan Tech 2014;24(3):e92–4.
35. Geyl S, Legros R, Charissou A, et al. Peroral endoscopic pyloromyotomy accelerates gastric emptying in healthy pigs: proof of concept. Endosc Int open 2016; 4(7):E796.
36. Jung Y, Lee J, Gromski MA, et al. Assessment of the length of myotomy in peroral endoscopic pyloromyotomy (G-POEM) using a submucosal tunnel technique (video). Surg Endosc 2015;29(8):2377–84.
37. Snape W, Lin M, Agarwal N, et al. Evaluation of the pylorus with concurrent intraluminal pressure and EndoFLIP in patients with nausea and vomiting. Neurogastroenterol Motil 2016;28(5):758–64.
38. Gourcerol G, Tissier F, Melchior C, et al. Impaired fasting pyloric compliance in gastroparesis and the therapeutic response to pyloric dilatation. Aliment Pharmacol Ther 2015;41(4):360–7.
39. Malik Z, Sankineni A, Parkman H. Assessing pyloric sphincter pathophysiology using EndoFLIP in patients with gastroparesis. Neurogastroenterol Motil 2015; 27(4):524–31.
40. Al-Bayati I, Sarosiek I, McCallum RW. Gastric electrical stimulation, pyloroplasty, gastrectomy, and acustimulation for the treatment of nausea and vomiting in the setting of gastroparesis. In: Koch K, Hasler W, editors. Nausea and vomiting. Cham(Switzerland): Springer; 2017.
41. McCallum RW, Snape W, Brody F, et al. Gastric electrical stimulation with Enterra therapy improves symptoms from diabetic gastroparesis in a prospective study. Clin Gastroenterol Hepatol 2010;8(11):947–54 [quiz: e116].

Printed and bound by CPI Group (UK) Ltd, Croydon, CR0 4YY

08/05/2025

01864739-0001